Essential Guide
to Blood Groups

Essential Guide to Blood Groups

SECOND EDITION

Geoff Daniels, PhD, FRCPath

Consultant Clinical Scientist
Bristol Institute for Transfusion Services
NHS Blood and Transplant
Bristol, UK

Imelda Bromilow, MSc, CBiol

General Manager
Scientific Services
Lateral Grifols Pty
Melbourne
Australia

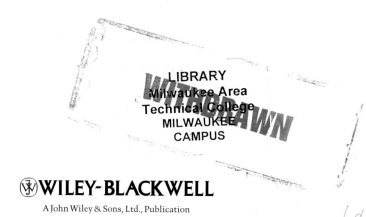
WILEY-BLACKWELL

A John Wiley & Sons, Ltd., Publication

This edition first published 2010, © 2007, 2010 by Geoff Daniels and Imelda Bromilow.

Blackwell Publishing was acquired by John Wiley & Sons in February 2007. Blackwell's publishing program has been merged with Wiley's global Scientific, Technical and Medical business to form Wiley-Blackwell.

Registered office: John Wiley & Sons Ltd, The Atrium, Southern Gate, Chichester, West Sussex, PO19 8SQ, UK

Editorial offices: 9600 Garsington Road, Oxford, OX4 2DQ, UK
The Atrium, Southern Gate, Chichester, West Sussex, PO19 8SQ, UK
111 River Street, Hoboken, NJ 07030-5774, USA

For details of our global editorial offices, for customer services and for information about how to apply for permission to reuse the copyright material in this book please see our website at www.wiley.com/wiley-blackwell

Library of Congress Cataloging-in-Publication Data
Daniels, Geoff.
    Essential guide to blood groups / Geoff Daniels, Imelda Bromilow. — 2nd ed.
        p. ; cm.
    Includes bibliographical references and index.
    ISBN 978-1-4443-3530-9
    1. Blood groups—Handbooks, manuals, etc. I. Bromilow, Imelda. II. Title.
    [DNLM: 1. Blood Group Antigens—Handbooks. WH 39 D186e 2010]
    QP91.D354 2010
    612.1′1825—dc22

                                                            2010010780

ISBN:978-1-44433530-9

A catalogue record for this book is available from the British Library.

Set in 9/12pt Palatino by Graphicraft Limited, Hong Kong
Printed and bound in the United States of America by Sheridan Books, Inc.

03 2012

Contents

Abbreviations

ADCC	antibody dependent cell-mediated cytotoxicity
AET	2-aminoethylisothiouronium bromide
AHG	anti-human globulin
AIHA	autoimmune haemolytic anaemia
AML	acute myeloid leukaemia
CAPA	corrective and preventive action
CGD	chronic granulomatous disease
CHAD	cold haemagglutinin disease
CLT	chemiluminescence test
CMV	cytomegalovirus
cv	co-efficient of variation
DAF	decay accelerating factor
DARC	Duffy antigen receptor for chemokines
DAT	direct antiglobulin test
DTT	dithiothreitol
EDTA	ethylenediaminetetraacetic acid
ETC	enzyme treated cells
FMH	feto-maternal haemorrhage
GP	glycophorin
GPI	glycosylphosphatidylinositol
HA	haemolytic anaemia
Hb	haemoglobin
HCT	haematocrit
HDFN	haemolytic disease of the fetus and newborn
HFA	high frequency antigen
HLA	human leucocyte antigen
HTR	haemolytic transfusion reaction
IAT	indirect antiglobulin test
ICAM	intercellular adhesion molecule
Ig	immunoglobulin
IL	interleukin
IS	immediate spin

ISBT	International Society of Blood Transfusion
IUT	intrauterine transfusions
LFA	low frequency antigen
LISS	low ionic strength saline
LW	Landsteiner–Wiener
MAC	membrane attack complex
MCA	middle cerebral artery
MGSA	melanoma growth stimulatory activity
MMA	monocyte monolayer assay
NANA	N-acetyl neuraminic acid
NISS	normal ionic strength saline
PBS	phosphate buffered saline
PCH	paroxysmal cold haemoglobinuria
PCR	polymerase chain reaction
PEG	polyethylene glycol
PNH	paroxysmal nocturnal haemoglobinuria
QA	quality assurance
QC	quality control
RBC	red blood cell
RCA	root cause analysis
SNP	single nucleotide polymorphism
SOP	standard operating procedure
TQM	total quality management
WAIHA	warm antibody immune haemolytic anaemia

An introduction to blood groups

CHAPTER 1

What is a blood group?

In 1900, Landsteiner showed that people could be divided into three groups (now called A, B, and O) on the basis of whether their red cells clumped when mixed with separated sera from other people. A fourth group (AB) was soon found. This is the origin of the term 'blood group'.

A blood group could be defined as, 'An inherited character of the red cell surface, detected by a specific alloantibody.' Do blood groups have to be present on red cells? This is the usual meaning, although platelet- and neutrophil-specific antigens might also be called blood groups. In this book only red cell surface antigens are considered. Blood groups do not have to be red cell-specific, or even blood cell-specific, and most are also detected on other cell types. Blood groups do have to be detected by a specific antibody: polymorphisms suspected of being present on the red cell surface, but only detected by other means, such as DNA sequencing, are not blood groups. Furthermore, the antibodies must be alloantibodies, implying that some individual lacks the blood group.

Blood group antigens may be:
- proteins;
- glycoproteins, with the antibody recognising primarily the polypeptide backbone;
- glycoproteins, with the antibody recognising the carbohydrate moiety;
- glycolipids, with the antibody recognising the carbohydrate portion.

Blood group polymorphisms may be as fundamental as representing the presence or absence of the whole macromolecule (e.g. RhD), or as minor as a single amino acid change (e.g. Fy^a and Fy^b) or a single monosaccharide difference (e.g. A and B).

Essential Guide to Blood Groups, 2nd edition. By Geoff Daniels and Imelda Bromilow. Published 2010 by Blackwell Publishing Ltd.

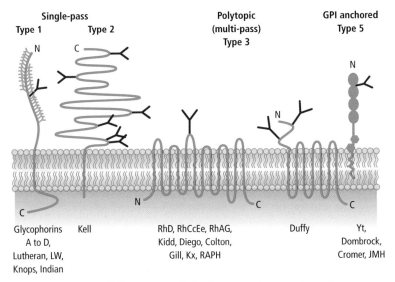

| Single-pass | | Polytopic | GPI anchored |
| Type 1 | Type 2 | (multi-pass)
Type 3 | Type 5 |

| Glycophorins
A to D,
Lutheran, LW,
Knops, Indian | Kell | RhD, RhCcEe, RhAG,
Kidd, Diego, Colton,
Gill, Kx, RAPH | Duffy | Yt,
Dombrock,
Cromer, JMH |

Fig. 1.1 Diagram of different types of blood group active proteins and glycoproteins, based on their integration into the red cell surface membrane. Listed are examples of blood group antigens for each type. (Type 4 proteins are cytoplasmic and not present in red cells.)

Blood group proteins and glycoproteins are integral structures of the red cell membrane. Diagrammatic representations of some blood group proteins and glycoproteins in the membrane are shown in Fig. 1.1. Some pass through the membrane once. These generally have an external N-terminal domain and a cytoplasmic C-terminal domain (Type 1), although in one case (the Kell glycoprotein) the C-terminus is external and the N-terminus internal (Type 2). Some are polytopic (Type 3); that is, they cross the membrane several times. Usually both termini are cytoplasmic, but the Duffy glycoprotein has an odd number of membrane-spanning domains and an extracellular N-terminal domain. Finally, some have no membrane-spanning domain, but are anchored to the membrane by a lipid tail (called a glycosylphosphatidylinositol or GPI anchor), which is attached to the C-terminus of the protein through carbohydrate (Type 5). There are no Type 4 glycoproteins, which have no external domain, in the red cell membrane.

Most red cell surface proteins are glycosylated, the only exceptions being the Rh and Kx proteins. This glycosylation may be (1) N-glycosylation, large, branched sugars attached to asparagine residues of the amino acid backbone, or (2) O-glycosylation, smaller glycans (usually tetrasaccharides) attached to serine or threonine residues.

Blood group antibodies

Blood groups are antigens and, by definition, a molecule cannot be an antigen unless it is recognised by an antibody (or T-cell receptor). So all blood group specificities are defined by antibodies. Most adults have antibodies to the A or B antigens, or to both; that is, they have 'naturally occurring' antibodies to those ABO antigens they lack. For most other blood groups corresponding antibodies are not 'naturally occurring', but are only formed as a result of immunisation by transfused red cells or by fetal red cells leaking into the maternal circulation during pregnancy or childbirth.

Blood group antibodies are usually IgM or IgG, although some may be IgA (see Chapter 6). 'Naturally occurring' antibodies are usually predominantly IgM, whereas 'immune' antibodies are predominantly IgG. As a general rule, IgM antibodies will directly agglutinate antigen-positive red cells in a saline medium, whereas most IgG antibodies require potentiators or anti-human globulin to effect agglutination (see Chapter 2).

Clinical importance of blood groups

Blood groups are of great clinical importance in blood transfusion and in transplantation. In fact, the discovery of the ABO system was one of the most important factors in making the practice of blood transfusion possible. Many blood group antibodies have the potential to cause rapid destruction of transfused red cells bearing the corresponding antigen, giving rise to a haemolytic transfusion reaction (HTR), either immediately or several days after the transfusion. At their worst, HTRs give rise to disseminated intravascular coagulation, renal failure, and death. At their mildest, they reduce the efficacy of the transfusion (see Chapter 6).

IgG blood group antibodies can cross the placenta during pregnancy and haemolyse fetal red cells expressing the corresponding antigen. This may cause alloimmune fetal haemolytic anaemia, more commonly known as haemolytic disease of the fetus and newborn (HDFN). Many blood group antibodies have the potential to cause HDFN, but the most common culprits are D and c of the Rh system and K of the Kell system.

Biological importance of blood groups

The biological importance of many blood group antigens is either known or can be surmised from their structure. The following functions have been attributed to blood group antigens: transporters of biologically important molecules across the red cell membrane; receptors of external stimuli and cell adhesion; regulators of autologous complement to prevent red cell destruction; enzymes; anchors of the red cell membrane to the cytoskeleton; and providers of an extracellular carbohydrate matrix to protect the cell from mechanical damage and microbial attack. Very little is known, however, about the functions of the blood group polymorphisms, but it is likely that they arose from selection pressures created by pathogens exploiting blood group molecules for attachment to the cells and subsequent invasion.

Blood group systems

The International Society of Blood Transfusion recognises 328 blood group antigens; 284 of these are classified into one of 30 blood group systems (Table 1.1 and see http://blood.co.uk/ibgrl/). Each blood group system represents either a single gene or a cluster of two or three closely linked genes of related sequence and with little or no recognised recombination occurring between them. Consequently, each blood group system is a genetically discrete entity. The MNS system comprises three genes, Rh, Xg, and Chido/Rodgers, two genes each, and each of the remainder represents a single gene. Rh and MNS are the most complex systems, with 52 and 46 antigens, respectively; eight systems consist of just a single antigen.

Blood group terminology and classification

Since the discovery of the ABO system in 1900, a multitude of blood group antigens have been identified and many different styles of terminology have been used. These include the following to represent alleles: upper case letters (e.g. A, B; M, N); upper and lower case letters to represent antithetical antigens, the products of alleles (S, s; K, k); superscript letters (Fy^a, Fy^b), and numbers (Lu6, Lu9). A variety of different styles of terminology have been used even within one system (e.g. Kell system: K, k; Kp^a, Kp^b, Kp^c; K12, K13).

In 1980, the International Society of Blood Transfusion (ISBT) established a Working Party to devise a genetically based numerical terminology for blood groups. This terminology is based on the blood group systems (Table 1.1). Each system has a three-digit number plus a 3–5 upper case letter symbol. For example, the Kell system is 006 or KEL (Table 1.2). Each antigen within that system has a three-digit number. K is 001 and Kp^a is 003, and so become 006001 or KEL1 and 006003 or KEL3, respectively. The full numerical symbol is seldom used and the alphanumerical symbols, with the redundant zeros removed, are more commonly employed. Phenotypes consist of the system symbol, followed by a colon, followed by a list of antigens shown to be present. Absent antigens

Table 1.1 The blood group systems

No.	Name	Symbol	No. of antigens	Gene name(s)*	CD No.	Chromo-some
001	ABO	ABO	4	*ABO*		9
002	MNS	MNS	46	*GYPA, GYPB, GYPE*	CD235	4
003	P1PK	P1	2	*P1*		22
004	Rh	RH	52	*RHD, RHCE*	CD240	1
005	Lutheran	LU	20	*LU* or *BCAM*	CD239	19
006	Kell	KEL	32	*KEL*	CD238	7
007	Lewis	LE	6	*LE* or *FUT3*		19
008	Duffy	FY	5	*FY* or *DARC*	CD234	1
009	Kidd	JK	3	*JK* or *SLC14A1*		18
010	Diego	DI	22	*DI* or *SLC4AE1*	CD233	17
011	Yt	YT	2	*YT* or *ACHE*		7
012	Xg	XG	2	*XG, CD99*	CD99	X/Y
013	Scianna	SC	7	*SC* or *ERMAP*		1
014	Dombrock	DO	7	*DO* or *ART4*	CD297	12
015	Colton	CO	4	*CO* or *AQP1*		7
016	Landsteiner–Wiener	LW	3	*LW* or *ICAM4*	CD242	19
017	Chido/Rodgers	CH/RG	9	*C4A, C4B*		6
018	H	H	1	*FUT1*	CD173	19
019	Kx	XK	1	*XK*		X
020	Gerbich	GE	11	*GE* or *GYPC*	CD236	2
021	Cromer	CROM	16	*CROM* or *CD55*	CD55	1
022	Knops	KN	9	*KN* or *CR1*	CD35	1
023	Indian	IN	4	*IN* or *CD44*	CD44	11
024	Ok	OK	3	*OK* or *BSG*	CD147	19
025	Raph	RAPH	1	*RAPH* or *CD151*	CD151	11
026	John Milton Hagen	JMH	6	*JMH* or *SEMA7A*	CD108	15
027	I	I	1	*I* or *GCNT2*		6
028	Globoside	GLOB	1	*B3GALT3*		3
029	Gill	GIL	1	*GIL* or *AQP3*		9
030	RHAG	RHAG	3	*RHAG*	CD241	6

*Where alternative gene names are given, the first is that of the ISBT, the second of the Human Genome Organisation.

are also listed, preceded by a minus symbol (Table 1.2). Genes have the system symbol followed by an asterisk, followed by the number of the antigen encoded by the allele.

For an antigen to join an existing blood group system there must be substantial evidence that it is encoded by the gene (or cluster of genes)

Table 1.2 Some examples of blood group terminology

	Original	Numerical
Antigen	K, k, Kp^a, Kp^b Co^a, Co^b	KEL1, KEL2, KEL3, KEL4 CO1, CO2
Phenotype	K− k+ Kp(a−b+) Jk(a−b+)	KEL: −1,2,−3,4 JK: −1,2
Gene	*K, k, Kp^a, Kp^b* *Fy^a, Fy^b*	*KEL*1, KEL*2, KEL*3, KEL*4* *FY*1, FY*2*
Genotype/haplotype	*kKp^b/kKp^b* *MS/Ms*	*KEL*2,4/2,4* *MNS*1,3/1,4*

producing the other antigens in the system. For one or more antigens to form a new system, they must be shown to be genetically discrete from all the existing systems.

Because the ISBT terminology is based on the blood groups systems, it functions as a blood group classification. It is not essential to use the numerical terminology. Indeed, it is not generally used in this book. It is, however, important to understand it, so as to understand the classification of blood groups.

Some blood group antigens have not been allocated to systems, owing to insufficient genetical evidence. If they are of low frequency, they are placed in the 700 Series of antigens, and if of high frequency, in the 901 Series. If two or more antigens are categorised together on the basis of genetical, serological, or biochemical information, but, due to lack of appropriate evidence, cannot be allocated to a system or form a new system, then they can form a blood group collection. The series and collections are described in Chapter 5.

Techniques used in blood grouping

Routine blood grouping still relies primarily on haemagglutination reactions between antigens and antibodies that are read and interpreted either manually or by automated means. The principles behind haemagglutination reactions, the discovery of the biochemistry of blood group antigens, and the increasing knowledge of the properties of immunoglobulins associated with blood group antibodies led to the development of laboratory tests other than direct agglutination. Antiglobulin methods and enzyme technology were introduced as routine methods for the detection of antigen–antibody reactions and played a part in the discovery and expansion of knowledge of blood group systems in general. Since these advances, non-routine methods have become available for specialist investigations and as research tools, such as flow cytometry and analysis of antigens at the molecular level.

Factors affecting antigen–antibody reactions

Temperature

The types of chemical bonds involved in a reaction are influenced by temperature. Polar (attractive) bonding in which electrons are interchanged between donor and acceptor molecules takes place in water-based media. The hydrogen bonds formed are exothermic and so stronger at lower temperatures. This type of bonding is normally associated with carbohydrate antigens.

Non-polar molecules form hydrophobic bonds by expelling water and occur at higher temperatures. They are associated with protein antigens.

The thermal range of an antibody is an indication of its clinical importance. Antibodies that promote accelerated red cell destruction *in vivo*, apart from antibodies of the ABO system, react optimally at 37°C

Essential Guide to Blood Groups, 2nd edition. By Geoff Daniels and Imelda Bromilow. Published 2010 by Blackwell Publishing Ltd.

(see Chapter 6). Large increases in temperature may have the effect of increasing the dissociation of the antigen–antibody complexes. This phenomenon is used in elution methods to free red cells of bound antibody, for example by heating to 56°C. For an antibody with an optimum temperature for reaction of 37°C, lowering the reaction temperature decreases the rate of association, necessitating a longer incubation time or alteration of other test parameters. However, antibodies with low avidity may react at 37°C but the antigen–antibody complexes dissociate rapidly. This dissociation may be minimised by reducing the temperature after sensitisation at 37°C has taken place.

Time and ionic strength

In order to speed up the interaction of antigen and antibody, the ionic strength of the test milieu can be lowered. This means that solutions of saline containing less Na^+ and Cl^- ions than normal isotonic salt solutions interfere less in the reaction between an antigen and antibody of complementary electrostatic charge. This is because the ions cluster around and neutralise the opposite charges on the antigen and antibody molecules. By reducing the numbers of free ions in solution, this 'neutralising' effect is diminished, thus enhancing the speed at which the antigen–antibody complexes are formed. Such solutions are known as low ionic strength saline (LISS). However, the reduction in ionic strength must be controlled to prevent non-specific uptake of immunoglobulins in 'sub-LISS' conditions.

pH

The optimal pH for most antibodies of clinical importance has not been determined; however, it is known that some antibodies react better at pHs other than the physiological pH range. Certain examples of anti-M react optimally at a pH of below 7 and in order to identify the specificity it may be necessary to acidify the serum. Under normal circumstances, a pH of about 7 is acceptable because red cells carry a negative charge and at pH 7–7.5 most antibody molecules bear a weakly positive charge. This enhances the attraction between the reactants during the first stage of agglutination or sensitisation. The use of phosphate buffered saline (PBS) ensures that the saline used in routine laboratory tests is not acidic. Significant lowering of the pH conditions increases dissociation of antigen–antibody complexes. This property is used to good effect in acid elution procedures in the laboratory, where it is desirable to dissociate the antibody from its antigen.

Antigen density

The number of antigen sites per cell and the accessibility of those antigens affects the optimal uptake of appropriate antibody. However, in conditions of antigen excess, the number of molecules of antibody bound on adjacent cells is relatively reduced, thereby producing less agglutination, or the formation of few, although large agglutinates. Antibody excess is therefore usually employed in routine test methods. The serum to cell ratio is therefore of importance in immunohaematological reactions. In LISS conditions, for example, the serum to cell ratio requires to be at a minimum ratio of 40 : 1. A lower ratio is associated with decreased test system sensitivity. The serum to cell ratio of a system can be found using the formula

$$\frac{(\text{Volume of serum} \times 100)}{(\text{Volume of cells}) \times (\% \text{ cell suspension})}$$

Thus, for a LISS technique using 2 volumes of serum and 2 volumes of cells at a 1.5% cell suspension, the serum to cell ratio ($2 \times 100 \div 2 \times 1.5\%$), would be about 66 : 1.

If the antibody has a low binding constant (K_o), increasing the amount of antibody enhances the test sensitivity but the prozone phenomenon may occur where an antibody is in excess and inhibits agglutination. This is because all available antigen sites are saturated by antibody, leaving no free sites for the formation of bridges by an antibody attached to another cell. Often, this situation can produce many, very small agglutinates or no visible agglutination at all. On dilution of the antibody, the reaction can proceed to normal agglutination strength, i.e. to the 'zone of equivalence' rather than the *pro*zone of antibody excess.

Stages of haemagglutination reactions

The first stage of a haemagglutination reaction is the formation of antigen–antibody complexes or sensitisation of the red cells by the antibody. In blood group serology, antibodies are most commonly one of two classes of immunoglobulins, IgG and IgM, although IgA antibodies with blood group specificity are known.

The red cell has a diameter of about 7–8 µm and IgG immunoglobulin a maximum dimension of about 14 nm with IgM molecules having a maximum distance of about 30 nm between antigen binding sites. To understand what this means, the red cell can be imagined as being 50 m wide with an IgG molecule as about 7 cm. Even though the IgM molecule is slightly larger, both classes of antibody have to attach to combining sites on more than one cell in order to promote haemagglutination, the second stage of the reaction. However, IgM molecules possess five times the number of combining sites than IgG and so can more readily cause direct agglutination of red cells. In order to promote agglutination by IgG antibodies, the test system generally requires to be enhanced, either to bring the red cells closer to each other so that the IgG molecules can bridge the gap between cells, or by using another antibody to attach to the IgG molecules producing agglutination. Thus, the second stage consists of either direct or indirect haemagglutination.

Direct agglutination

As the name suggests, this occurs as a direct result of an antigen–antibody interaction. Generally, the antibody is of the IgM immunoglobulin class and reactions take place optimally at low temperatures. Examples of IgG antibodies that can effect direct agglutination are known, such as anti-A and anti-B, and some IgG class anti-M. This is thought to be due to the structure carrying the appropriate antigen extending above the red cell surface so that the distance between antigens on adjacent cells is less than 14 nm. This is the minimum distance between adjacent cells under normal conditions of ionic concentration, due to the mutual repulsive affect of the negative charge associated with red blood cells. An IgG molecule can therefore cross-link the two cells and produce agglutination. IgM antibodies can span a larger distance, have more antigen binding capacity and are associated more readily with direct agglutination. Antigen site density can also influence the reaction, as the more antigen sites per cell, the better the chance of antigen–antibody complex formation and subsequent agglutination. Proximity of antigens on a cell does not necessarily promote agglutination because one antibody molecule may bind to antigens on the same cell, thus preventing the formation of bridges between two cells, necessary for agglutination.

In the routine laboratory, most direct agglutination techniques are used in ABO forward and reverse grouping tests or in the determination of other red cell antigens with human, polyclonal or monoclonal, directly agglutinating antibodies. These tests can be performed on slides, in tubes, by solid/liquid phase microplate technology, or by using a column agglutination technique, without the necessity of enhancing the reaction in order to visualise the haemagglutination. However, slide techniques are not recommended for initial or definitive antigen determinations, particularly when dealing with neonatal samples, as certain blood group antigens may not be fully developed at birth. The use of a relatively insensitive technique can therefore lead to mis-typing in some cases.

Some antibodies can initiate the complement cascade (Fig. 2.1) through to the membrane attack complex (MAC), leading to haemolysis of the red cells. This may be mistaken for a negative result in laboratory tests but is actually positive. For reverse ABO grouping, ethylenediaminetetraacetic acid (EDTA) anti-coagulated samples are used to prevent this, or reagent

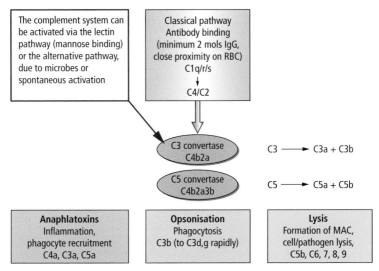

Fig. 2.1 Complement activation may be initiated by antibody binding to the appropriate antigens on the red blood cells (RBC). IgM antibodies activate complement very efficiently and often initiate the complement cascade through to the membrane attack complex (MAC), with subsequent lysis of the cells. IgG antibodies require a minimum of two molecules in close proximity on the red cell for initiation of complement activation, generally only up to the C3 stage.

cells suspended in EDTA saline for serum samples. The EDTA prevents the complement activation after the C1q stage by chelating Ca^{2+} ions required for the cascade to continue.

Indirect agglutination

Antibodies that cannot directly agglutinate cells are detected by means of enhanced test systems, notably the use of enzyme treatment of red cells or by the antiglobulin test.

Enzyme techniques

Enzymes often used in blood group serology are the proteases bromelin, ficin and papain, which have broad specificity for peptide bonds, and trypsin and chymotrypsin, which have more precise specificities. Neuraminidase, which cleaves sialic acid residues, is the most effective enzyme at reducing the surface charge of a red cell, but exposes the cryptantigen T. T-activated red cells are agglutinated by the naturally occurring T antibodies present in all normal human sera. Proteases also remove sialic acid residues attached to peptides and are generally used

Table 2.1 Some effects of enzyme treatment of red cells			
Cleavage of glycoprotein from the red cell membrane **Effect 1**	Carries sialic acid (NANA)*, major contributor to red cell-negative charge →	Reduces net negative charge →	Allows cells to be in closer contact, for antibody molecules to bridge the gap
Cleavage of glycoprotein from the red cell membrane **Effect 2**	Glycoproteins are hydrophilic (attract water molecules) →	Water molecules need to be shared by neighbouring red cells →	Makes red cells come into closer contact with each other
Cleavage of glycoprotein from the red cell membrane **Effect 3**	Glycoprotein structures protrude from the red cell membrane surface →	Reduced steric hindrance →	Antigens more readily accessible to antibodies
Cleavage of glycoprotein from the red cell membrane **Effect 4**	Carries certain red cell antigens →	Antigens lost, notably M, N, S, and Duffy system →	Antibodies of these specificities undetected

*NANA, N-acetyl neuraminic acid or sialic acid.

because they are more effective at increasing the ability of certain antibodies to promote agglutination. These proteases do not usually cause T activation. The effects of protease treatment of red cells are listed in Table 2.1.

Enzyme-treated cells are used in antibody screening and, importantly, in antibody identification procedures. They are particularly useful for determining specificities within mixtures of antibodies, where one or more are directed against enzyme-sensitive antigens.

Enzyme methods are difficult to standardise. Traditionally, enzyme solutions were prepared using a weight-for-volume method. However, not all powder forms of an enzyme will contain the same amount of activity and it is necessary to analyse each prepared batch for activity to ensure standardised tests. The red cell papainisation procedure should also be carefully monitored and controlled to prevent over-sensitisation, resulting in the exposure of cryptantigens, such as the T antigen.

Antiglobulin tests

Carlo Moreschi first described the principle of the antiglobulin technique in 1908. However, it was Coombs, Mourant and Race who introduced the antiglobulin test into routine laboratory practice. Coombs and his co-workers showed that the test could be used to detect blood group antibodies in serum, the indirect antiglobulin test (IAT; Fig. 2.2) or to demonstrate the sensitisation of red cells *in vivo*, the direct antiglobulin test (DAT; Fig. 2.3).

In polyspecific anti-human globulin (AHG) only anti-IgG and anti-C3d are required. For automated procedures, which require the use of anti-coagulated samples, only anti-IgG is used for the detection of antibodies of potential clinical importance. Antibodies that depend on the detection of complement components on the red cell without concomitant IgG, are rare.

There is a correlation between the number of bound IgG molecules and the strength of a reaction in the IAT and the DAT. The minimum number of bound molecules for detection is in the region of 100–150. As this figure

Indirect antiglobulin test

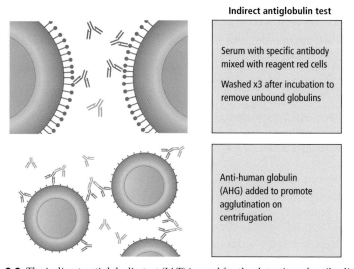

Serum with specific antibody mixed with reagent red cells

Washed x3 after incubation to remove unbound globulins

Anti-human globulin (AHG) added to promote agglutination on centrifugation

Fig. 2.2 The indirect antiglobulin test (IAT) is used for the detection of antibodies of the IgG class. In spin-tube techniques, unbound immunoglobulins or other protein is washed from the test system and anti-human globulin (AHG) is added to the sensitised cells. During centrifugation the AHG promotes agglutination and thus visible haemagglutination. The IAT is used for identification of antibody(ies) in the serum and/or plasma of a potential transfusion recipient or as part of antenatal testing, to help to assess the likelihood of the antibody promoting fetal red cell destruction. It can also be used with known antibodies for typing antigens on the red cell.

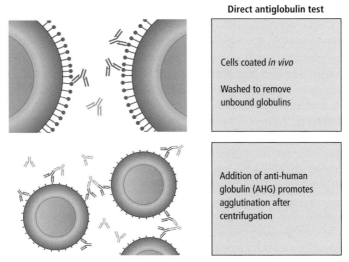

Direct antiglobulin test

Cells coated *in vivo*

Washed to remove unbound globulins

Addition of anti-human globulin (AHG) promotes agglutination after centrifugation

Fig. 2.3 The direct antiglobulin test (DAT) is used for the demonstration of *in vivo* sensitisation of red cells with immunoglobulin and/or complement. This can occur after antigen–antibody complexes have been formed, for example in certain disease states such as autoimmune haemolytic anaemia (AIHA) or haemolytic disease of the fetus and newborn (HDFN). The DAT may also be positive following a transfusion of antigen positive blood, to which the recipient possesses the antibody.

increases, so does the strength of reaction up to maximum agglutination strength achieved between 500 and 2000 molecules per cell.

Variations on the original normal ionic strength saline (NISS) antiglobulin test exist, the most useful being the LISS method, introduced in the 1970s by Löw and Messeter. Lowering the ionic strength of the saline increases the speed of uptake of antibody. This allows the incubation time for IAT procedures to be reduced to 15 minutes. An IAT may be performed by LISS addition or with the reagent cells suspended in LISS. In LISS techniques, the serum to cell ratio is critical. Increasing the volume of serum has the effect of decreasing the sensitivity of the test, as the addition of the serum raises the final ionic strength of the test system and lowers the rate of antibody uptake.

Antiglobulin techniques are used for antibody screening and identification and for serological cross-matching, to detect incompatibility caused by an IgG antibody of potential clinical importance that was not detected during screening (see Chapter 6).

Other techniques include the use of polyethylene glycol (PEG) to enhance the detection of weak antibodies. Anti-IgG should be used alone

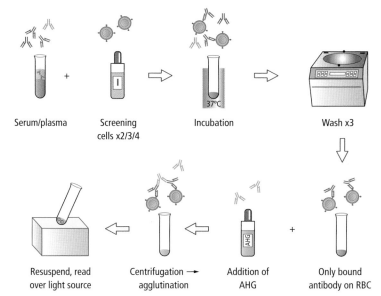

| Serum/plasma | Screening cells x2/3/4 | Incubation | Wash x3 |

| Resuspend, read over light source | Centrifugation → agglutination | Addition of AHG | Only bound antibody on RBC |

Fig. 2.4 Principle of indirect antiglobulin test: spin-tube method. The conventional 'spin-tube' method for the IAT entails washing the cells after incubation. This is an important part of the procedure, as a poor wash phase may leave residual human globulin that can neutralise the added AHG. This would result in a falsely weak or negative result. All IAT methods that require a wash phase should incorporate control of apparent negatives with pre-sensitised cells after reading and recording the result. The control should be positive, demonstrating that the AHG has not been neutralised and the test is truly negative. The completed test is usually read macroscopically, over a light source after gentle agitation to resuspend the cell button.

for this method, as the red cells take up complement non-specifically when suspended in PEG medium.

Antiglobulin tests were initially performed on well-scrubbed tiles, with reconstituted freeze-dried AHG. The method was advanced with the advent of the spin-tube technique (Fig. 2.4) and, subsequently, solid phase microplate methods were introduced (Fig. 2.5). All of these methods require a wash phase and validation of negative reactions with IgG-coated red cells. In the 1980s, Yves Lapierre discovered a gel method to capture haemagglutination, which was developed by DiaMed AG. A LISS IAT method was devised that eliminated the wash phase and so reduced the potential for error associated with a poor wash technique, as well as contributing to laboratory standardisation and economy of effort (Fig. 2.6). The 'No-wash' technique is possible because, on centrifugation, the liquid phase of the reactants remains in the upper chamber of

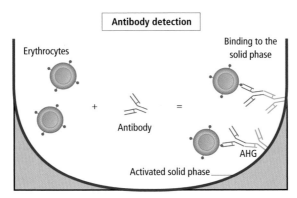

Fig. 2.5 The solid phase microplate method for the IAT has the AHG bound to the well of the microplate. Antibody bound to red cells bind to the solid phase AHG and haemagglutination is observed after unbound globulins are washed free.

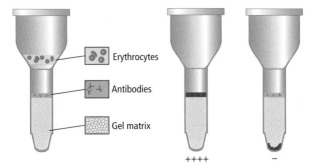

Fig. 2.6 Principle of the gel test. The 'No-wash' ID-System (gel column) for the IAT incorporates the AHG within the gel matrix. Sensitised cells react with the AHG on centrifugation, leaving the liquid reactants, including any unbound globulins in the reaction chamber. Cells free from IgG and/or complement components are centrifuged to the bottom of the microtube. No control of negative results is necessary as no washing is required.

the microtube and only the cells enter the gel matrix, which contains the AHG. Cells sensitised during the incubation phase react with the AHG and the agglutinates are held at the top of, or throughout, the gel matrix. Non-sensitised cells form a pellet at the base of the microtube. Because no liquid enters the gel, there is no danger of neutralisation of the AHG, which can happen in a spin-tube method owing to residual human proteins not removed during the wash phase. Weak positive reactions are also more robust in column agglutination techniques (CAT), there is no possibility of dissociation of the antigen–antibody complexes during a too-vigorous wash phase.

The sensitivity of antibody detection is, however, still affected by a number of other variables. The serum to cell ratio for a LISS IAT must be at least 40 : 1. The period of incubation must be sufficient to allow maximum uptake of antibody and depends on the binding constant of the antibody as well as the concentrations of antibody and antigen. Some weak antibodies may therefore need a longer time to react optimally, or an altered serum to cell ratio. Such adjustments to the basic technique are usually only employed in doubtful cases, or when samples are referred to a specialist laboratory for in-depth investigations. A reference laboratory may use a two-stage antiglobulin test, with the addition of fresh serum to provide complement to aid the detection of certain antibodies, notably in the Lewis and Kidd systems and for anti-Vel. Another non-routine IAT, which can be helpful particularly for the detection of Kidd antibodies, is the enzyme-antiglobulin test. In this method, the serum is tested against enzyme-treated cells and is then subject to an IAT.

Elution techniques

A subsidiary test that may be performed in the elucidation of weak antigens, separation of mixtures of antibodies, causative antibody in haemolytic disease of the fetus and newborn (HDFN), investigation of a transfusion reaction or the specificity of an autoantibody in autoimmune haemolytic anaemia (AIHA; see Chapter 6) is an elution technique.

Where an antigen is suspected to be present, but cannot be demonstrated by routine methods, the cells are incubated with appropriate antibody and the antibody subsequently eluted from the cells and identified. For example, this technique is required for detection of some very low subgroups of A, especially A_{el}, and for the very weak D antigen, DEL.

An eluate, the product of an elution procedure, can be obtained by using heat, organic solvents such as ether, or by reducing the pH. The eluate can then be subjected to identification procedures.

In performing an elution, an antibody may be identified in an eluate prepared with cells that are antigen-negative for that antibody. It is thought that this may be due to the non-specific uptake of IgG rather than to an 'unexpected' antibody. So-called 'mimicking' antibodies with apparent specificity (e.g. anti-C) are absorbed by antigen-negative as well as antigen-positive cells.

Automation of test procedures

Most laboratories today have tried to automate as many procedures as possible. This is mainly because of cost restraints and the attempt to promote further standardisation with fewer possibilities for error. Positive sample identification and data capture are therefore of prime importance. Automation also contributes to laboratory safety in that workers are less exposed to hazards from potentially infectious material.

For all serological testing requirements, there are several systems well established that employ microplate technology and/or column agglutination technology. The choice of automation depends upon the technology routinely in use, the throughput required, and the number and skill mix of laboratory staff.

Flow cytometry

Although not used as an automated system for routine typing of blood samples, flow cytometry can be applied in special circumstances; for example, when investigating the cause of double cell populations or for identifying weakly expressed antigens. It can also be used to assess the amount of feto-maternal haemorrhage (FMH) in RhD-negative mothers who require anti-D prophylaxis and for calculating the concentration of anti-D in an immunised RhD-negative antenatal woman.

The principle of flow cytometry is shown in Fig. 2.7. Basically, cells are incubated with antibodies conjugated with fluorophores, dyes that fluoresce under intense light. In the flow cytometer the cells pass, in single file, past a laser beam and fluorescence is monitored by photodetectors.

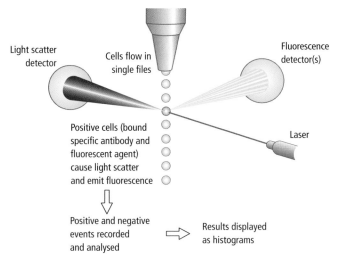

Fig. 2.7 Simplified diagram of the concept of flow cytometry, showing light scatter detector for forward and side scatter which indicate size and shape of the cells and one detector of fluorescence. More than one fluorescence detector is very often incorporated in order to visualise different 'events'.

As most flow cytometers can detect light of different wavelengths emitted by two or more different fluorophores, more than one antigen can be detected at the same time.

Flow cytometry enables large numbers of cells or 'events' to be examined in a short space of time. Its sensitivity is such that a small number of rare events can be detected accurately, if a sufficient number of total events are counted. This is because the cells arrive at the point of analysis in a random fashion and a sub-set of cells will also be randomly distributed within the suspension. To ensure precision, therefore, enough events must be recorded to allow the rare events to be detected. For example, if the number of fetal cells is in reality only 0.01% of the maternal sample, then at least 10^7 events or cells must be counted in total to give an accurate result, with an acceptable co-efficient of variation (cv).

Molecular blood group genotyping

All the clinically significant blood group polymorphisms are now understood at the molecular level, enabling techniques to be designed to predict blood group genotype from the DNA sequence. The technology is described in Chapter 7.

The ABO blood groups

CHAPTER 3

Introduction

The science of blood group serology materialised in 1900 with the discovery of the ABO blood groups by Landsteiner. Together with the development of anticoagulants, it was this discovery that made the practice of blood transfusion possible. Landsteiner mixed serum and red cells from different individuals and found that in some tests the cells were agglutinated (clumped) and in others they were not, demonstrating individual variation. The mixing of serum, or at least antibodies, with red cells followed by observation of the presence or absence of agglutination is the basis for most methods for determining blood group phenotype in use today. By 1910 the ABO blood groups had been shown to be inherited characters, in the 1950s they were shown to represent oligosaccharide chains on glycoproteins and glycolipids, and in 1990 the gene encoding the enzymes responsible for synthesis of the ABO antigens was cloned.

ABO is considered a blood group system because it was discovered on red cells and its antigens are readily detected, by haemagglutination techniques, on red cells. However, they are also present in many different tissues and organs, and in soluble form in secretions, and so are often referred to as histo-blood group antigens.

ABO antigens, antibodies, and inheritance

At its simplest, the ABO system consists of two antigens, A and B, the indirect products of the *A* and *B* alleles of the *ABO* gene (Table 3.1). A third allele, *O*, produces no antigen and is recessive to *A* and *B*. There are four phenotypes: A, B, AB, and O. The A phenotype results from the genotypes *A/A* or *A/O*, B phenotype from *B/B* or *B/O*, AB from *A/B*, and

---

Essential Guide to Blood Groups, 2nd edition. By Geoff Daniels and Imelda Bromilow.
Published 2010 by Blackwell Publishing Ltd.

Table 3.1 ABO antigens, antibodies, and genotypes

ABO group	Antigens on red cells	Antibodies in serum	Genotype
O	None	Anti-A,B	*O/O*
A	A	Anti-B	*A/A* or *A/O*
B	B	Anti-A	*B/B* or *B/O*
AB	A and B	None	*A/B*

O from *O/O*. Although many variations of the ABO phenotypes exist, almost all are basically quantitative modifications of the A and B antigens.

Landsteiner's rule states that individuals lacking A or B antigen from their red cells have the corresponding antibody in their plasma. In this respect, ABO is unique among blood group polymorphisms. Violations of Landsteiner's rule in adults are rare.

A_1 and A_2

The A phenotype can be subdivided into A_1 and A_2. A_1 is the more common phenotype in all populations. A_1 and A_1B red cells have a stronger expression of A antigen than A_2 and A_2B, respectively. With most anti-A reagents, A_1 red cells agglutinate faster, give a stronger agglutinate, and are agglutinated by higher dilutions of anti-A, than A_2 cells. Estimated numbers of antigens sites per red cell can be summarised as follows: A_1, $8–12 \times 10^5$; A_2, $1–4 \times 10^5$; A_1B, $5–9 \times 10^5$; A_2B, 1×10^5.

In addition to this quantitative dichotomy, there is also a qualitative difference between A_1 and A_2. About 2% of A_2 and 25% of A_2B individuals produce an antibody, called anti-A_1, that reacts with A_1 and A_1B cells, but not with A_2 or A_2B cells. The usual serological interpretation of this is that both A_1 and A_2 cells have A antigen, but A_1 cells have an additional antigen, called A_1, absent from A_2 cells (Table 3.2). Some lectins, which are sugar-binding proteins of non-immune and non-human origin, agglutinate

Table 3.2 A_1 and A_2 phenotypes

Phenotype	Anti-A (group B serum)	Anti-A_1 (group A_2 or A_2B serum)	*Dolichos biflorus* (suitably diluted)
A_1	+++	++	+++
A_2	++	0	0
A_1B	+++	++	++
A_2B	+	0	0

red cells. Appropriately diluted lectin from the seeds of *Dolichos biflorus*, an Indian legume, is a very effective anti-A_1 reagent, agglutinating A_1 and A_1B cells, but not A_2 or A_2B cells (Table 3.2).

Antigen, phenotype, and gene frequencies

The four phenotypes – A, B, O, and AB – are present in most populations, but their frequencies differ substantially throughout the world (Fig. 3.1). Phenotype, gene, and genotype frequencies for an indigenous British population are provided in Table 3.3.

Populations with a group O phenotype frequency greater than 60% are found in native people of the Americas and in parts of Africa and

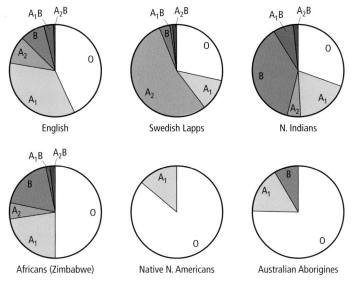

Fig. 3.1 A_1A_2BO phenotype frequencies in six selected populations.

Table 3.3 A_1A_2BO frequencies (%) in an indigenous British population

Phenotype		Gene		Genotype	
O	47	O	68	O/O	46.7
A	42	A	26	A/A	6.6
				A/O	35.1
B	8	B	6	B/B	0.3
				B/O	8.2
AB	3			A/B	3.1

Australia, but not in most of Europe or Asia. Some native people of South and Central America are virtually all group O, and probably were entirely so before the arrival of Europeans. The frequency of A is quite high (40–60%) in Europe, especially in Scandinavia and parts of Central Europe. Relatively high A frequency is also found in the Aborigines of South Australia (up to 77%) and in certain Native American tribes where the frequency reaches 50%. A_2 is found mainly in Europe, the Near East, and Africa, but is either very rare or absent from indigenous populations throughout the rest of the world. High frequencies of B are found in Central Asia (about 40%). In Europe, B frequency varies between 8% and 12%.

ABO antibodies

Anti-A and -B are almost invariably present when the corresponding antigen is absent. With the exception of newborn infants, deviations from this rule are rare. Missing antibodies may indicate a weak subgroup of A or B, chimerism, hypogammaglobulinaemia, or, occasionally, old age. ABO antibodies detected in the sera of neonates are usually IgG and maternal in origin, but are rarely IgM and produced by the fetus. Generally, ABO agglutinins are first detected at an age of about 3 months and continue to increase in titre, reaching adult levels between 5 and 10 years. Although ABO antibodies are often referred to as 'naturally occurring', they probably appear in children as a result of immunisation by A and B substances present in the environment.

Changes in the characteristics of anti-A or -B occur as a result of further immunisation by pregnancy or by artificial means, such as incompatible transfusion of red cells or other blood products. Typical serologically detectable changes are increase in titre and avidity of the agglutinin, increase in haemolytic activity, and greater activity at 37°C.

Anti-A and -B molecules may be IgM, IgG or IgA; some sera may contain all three classes. Anti-A and -B of non-stimulated individuals are predominantly IgM, although IgG and IgA may be present. IgG2 and IgG1 anti-A and -B are predominant, with IgG3 and IgG4 having a minor role.

Sera from group O people do not simply contain two separable antibodies, anti-A and -B, but a cross-reacting antibody called anti-A,B, which recognises a structure common to both A and B determinants. Anti-A,B molecules are mostly IgG, but may be IgM or IgA.

Numerous examples of monoclonal ABO antibodies have been produced, mostly in hybridomas of murine myeloma cells and lymphocytes of mice immunised with ABO substances or with red cells. Monoclonal anti-A and -B have proved to be very satisfactory reagents and are generally the reagents of choice, both for manual and automated techniques.

Importance of the ABO system to transfusion and transplantation medicine

ABO is the most important blood group system in transfusion medicine, because transfusion of ABO incompatible red cells will almost always result in symptoms of a haemolytic transfusion reaction (HTR) and can cause disseminated intravascular coagulation, renal failure, and death. Two types of ABO incompatibility can be distinguished.

- Major incompatibility, where antibodies in the recipient will destroy transfused red cells (e.g. A to O, B to O, A to B, B to A).
- Minor incompatibility, where antibodies in the donated blood will destroy the recipient's red cells (e.g. O to A, O to B).

Major incompatibility in blood transfusion must be avoided. Although minor incompatibility can usually be disregarded when the donor does not have exceptionally high levels of ABO antibodies, whenever possible donor blood of the same ABO group of that of the patient should be used for transfusion. Signs of red cell destruction may be apparent following transfusion of group O whole blood or, in exceptional circumstances, packed red cells, to recipients of other ABO groups. This is the result of destruction of the patient's red cells by transfused ABO antibodies. Anti-A$_1$ is rarely clinically significant and most examples are not active above 25°C, although there are a few reports of HTRs caused by anti-A$_1$.

IgG anti-A, -B, and -A,B are all capable of causing haemolytic disease of the fetus and newborn (HDFN), although HDFN caused by ABO antibodies is uncommon and almost only occurs in A$_1$, B, or A$_1$B babies of group O mothers. Despite the presence of IgG ABO antibodies in the serum of most group O women, severe ABO HDFN is rare for two main reasons: (1) fetal red cells have a relatively low density of A and B antigens; (2) soluble A and B substances are present in fetal plasma and other body fluids and can neutralise maternal antibodies. The complement deficiency of fetal plasma may also play a part in the rarity of ABO HDFN.

ABO antibodies can cause hyperacute rejection of incompatible kidney, liver, and heart transplants, but can usually be disregarded for tissue transplants, including cornea, skin, and bone. Successful major ABO-incompatible solid organ transplants are often achieved following reduction of ABO antibody levels in the plasma. Haemopoietic stem cells do not express ABO antigens, so ABO is often disregarded when selecting a stem cell donor. However, major ABO incompatibility may lead to haemolysis of infused red cells with a bone marrow transplant and can give rise to pure red cell aplasia and delayed red cell chimerism in non-myeloablative stem cell transplants.

The appearance of apparent autoanti-A or -B following transplantation of minor incompatible solid organs (e.g. O organ to A recipient) results from the presence of lymphoreticular tissue transplanted with the organ: passenger lymphocyte syndrome. Typically, these antibodies are IgG, appear 5–15 days after transplantation, and last for up to 3 months. They are often responsible for haemolysis and have caused acute renal failure and even death. Haemolysis induced by antibodies of graft origin may also be a complication of minor ABO incompatibility in stem cell transplantation.

Biochemical nature of the ABO antigens

A and B antigens are oligosaccharides. The most abundant structures on red cells carrying ABO activity are the N-linked oligosaccharides of red cell surface glycoproteins, predominantly the red cell anion exchanger (AE1, the Diego blood group antigen, or band 3) and the glucose transporter (GLUT1), although some other glycoproteins are also involved. ABO-active oligosaccharides are also present on glycolipids.

Oligosaccharides are chains of monosaccharide sugars: D-glucose (Glc); D-galactose (Gal); D-mannose (Man); N-acetyl-D-glucosamine (GlcNAc); N-acetyl-D-galactosamine (GalNAc); L-fucose (Fuc). An oligosaccharide is A-active when the terminal monosaccharide is GalNAc, in $\alpha1\rightarrow3$ linkage to a Gal residue that also has Fuc in $\alpha1\rightarrow2$ linkage, whereas an oligosaccharide is B-active when the terminal monosaccharide is Gal, in $\alpha1\rightarrow3$ linkage to the $\alpha1,2$-fucosylated Gal residue (Fig. 3.2). GalNAc and Gal are the immunodominant sugars of A and B antigens, respectively. Group O red cells lack both GalNAc and Gal from the $\alpha1,2$-fucosylated Gal residue (Fig. 3.2), so express neither A nor B. The A and B trisaccharides may be attached to several different core oligosaccharide chains, but in red cells the fucosylated Gal residue is usually in $\beta1\rightarrow4$ linkage to GlcNAc (Fig. 3.2). This is called a type 2 core structure. Less abundant core structures, called type 3 and type 4, are only present on glycolipids and may

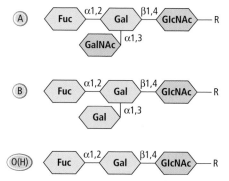

Fig. 3.2 Diagrammatic representation of A- and B-active oligosaccharides, plus the H-active oligosaccharide, the precursor of A and B. R, remainder of molecule.

also be involved A and B activity. Presence of type 4 structures on A_1 phenotype red cells, but not on A_2 cells, may account for the qualitative differences between A_1 and A_2.

Biosynthesis of the ABO antigens and ABO molecular genetics

Oligosaccharides are built up by the stepwise addition of monosaccharides. The addition of each monosaccharide requires a specific transferase, an enzyme that catalyses the transfer of the monosaccharide from its donor substrate, a nucleotide molecule carrying the relevant monosaccharide, to its acceptor substrate, the non-reducing end of the growing oligosaccharide chain. A-transferase, the product of the *A* allele, is a GalNAc-transferase, which catalyses the transfer of GalNAc from UDP-GalNAc (donor) to the fucosylated Gal residue (acceptor) (Fig. 3.3). B-transferase, the product of the *B* allele, is a Gal-transferase, which catalyses the transfer of Gal from UDP-Gal to the fucosylated Gal residue of the acceptor (Fig. 3.3). The *O* allele produces no active enzyme, and so the fucosylated Gal residue remains unsubstituted (and expresses H antigen).

The genetic basis for oligosaccharide blood groups is fundamentally different from that of the protein blood groups. Protein antigens are encoded directly by the blood group genes, but the genes governing carbohydrate polymorphism encode the transferase enzymes that catalyse

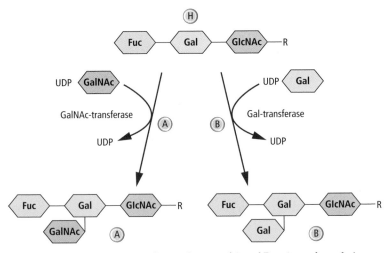

Fig. 3.3 Biosynthetic pathways for production of A and B antigens from their precursor (H).

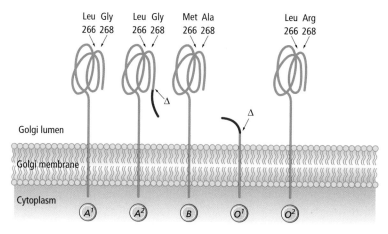

Fig. 3.4 Model of glycosyltransferase products of five alleles of *ABO*, showing the positions of the amino acid substitutions that are most important in determining the specificity of the enzymes. Δ, the position of the single nucleotide deletion in the A^2 and O^1 alleles that introduces a reading frameshift.

the biosynthesis of the blood group antigens. *A* and *B* alleles of the *ABO* gene encode the A- and B-transferases. These two enzymes differ by four amino acids, two of which (positions 266 and 268) are important in determining whether the enzyme has GalNAc-transferase (A) or Gal-transferase (B) activity (Fig. 3.4). The most common form of *O* allele (O^1) has the same sequence as A^1, apart from a deletion of a single nucleotide in the part of the gene encoding the stem of the enzyme. This disrupts the three-nucleotide amino acid code and also introduces a code for termination of translation of the mRNA. Consequently, the O^1 allele encodes a truncated protein, which could have no enzyme activity (Fig. 3.4). The product of another, much less common form of *O* allele, O^2, has a single amino acid change at position 268, introducing a charged arginine residue that disrupts the catalytic site and results in either no enzyme activity or possibly trace A-transferase activity (Fig. 3.4).

The *ABO* gene has seven exons. The amino acid substitutions that determine transferase specificity (A or B) are encoded by nucleotide polymorphisms in exon 7. The nucleotide deletion characteristic of O^1 alleles is in exon 6.

The A^2 allele has a single nucleotide deletion in exon 7 immediately before the position of the codon giving the instruction for termination of translation. This prevents translation termination at that position, resulting in a protein of extended length, which still has A-transferase activity, but is less efficient than the A_1-transferase (Fig. 3.4).

H, the precursor of A and B

An antigen called H is present on the red cells of almost everybody, but is expressed much more strongly on group O and A_2 cells than on A_1 and B cells. H is the biosynthetic precursor of A and B; the fucosylated Gal structure that is converted to the A-active trisaccharide by addition of GalNAc or to the B-active trisaccharide by addition of Gal (Figs 3.3 and 3.4). In group O individuals the H antigen remains unconverted and is expressed strongly. In A_1 and B individuals most of the H antigens are converted to A or B structures, but in A_2 individuals, in whom the A-transferase is less efficient than in A_1, many H-active structures remain.

The ultimate enzyme in the biosynthesis of H on red cells is a fucosyl-transferase (FucT1), which catalyses the fucosylation of the Gal residue of the H precursor (Fig. 3.5). *FUT1*, the gene encoding this fucosyltrans-ferase, is genetically independent of *ABO*; *FUT1* is on chromosome 19, *ABO* is on chromosome 9. ABO and H are, therefore, separate blood group systems. Very rare phenotypes exist in which homozygosity for mutations in *FUT1* results in no H being present on the red cells and consequently no A or B antigens are expressed on the red cells regardless of *ABO* genotype (see below).

ABH secretion

In addition to their presence on red cells, A, B, and H antigens are widely distributed in the body and in most people are present as soluble glyco-proteins in body secretions. A genetic polymorphism determines whether H antigen, and consequently A and B antigens, are present in secretions.

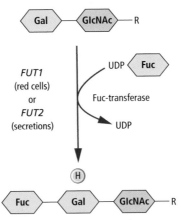

Fig. 3.5 Biosynthetic pathway for the production of H, the precursor of A and B.

Table 3.4 Haemagglutination-inhibition tests to determine ABH secretor status from saliva

	Anti-A + Saliva + A cells	Anti-B + Saliva + B cells	Anti-H* + Saliva + O cells
A secretor	Neg	Pos	Neg
B secretor	Pos	Neg	Neg
AB secretor	Neg	Neg	Neg
O secretor	Pos	Pos	Neg
Non-secretor (all ABO groups)	Pos	Pos	Pos

Ulex europaeus lectin.

About 80% of Caucasians are ABH-secretors: their secretions contain A plus a little H if they are group A, B plus some H if they are group B, and an abundance of H if they are group O. Secretions of ABH-non-secretors, who represent about 20% of the population, contain no H and, consequently, neither A nor B.

Secretor phenotypes are usually determined by detecting ABH substances in saliva by haemagglutination-inhibition techniques. Boiled saliva is mixed with anti-A, -B, and -H reagents and group A, B, and O red cells, respectively, are added to the mixtures (Table 3.4). Lectin from the seeds of common gorse, *Ulex europaeus*, is generally used as an anti-H reagent. In secretors, the soluble blood group substance will bind to the antibody or lectin and block agglutination of the appropriate indicator cell. In non-secretors, the antibodies are not blocked and agglutination occurs.

The enzyme responsible for synthesis of H antigen on red cells is a fucosyltransferase produced by the *FUT1* gene. This gene is active in mesodermally derived tissues, which includes the haemopoietic tissue responsible for production of red cells. *FUT1* is not active in endodermally derived tissues, which are responsible for body secretions such as saliva. Another gene, *FUT2*, which produces a fucosyltransferase (FucT2) very similar to that produced by *FUT1*, is active in endodermally derived tissues, so *FUT2* controls secretion of H. Homozygosity for inactivating mutations in *FUT2* are responsible for the non-secretor phenotype. Such inactivating mutations are common in *FUT2*. The most common Caucasian *FUT2* inactivating mutation converts the codon for tryptophan-143 to a translation stop codon. In group A and B non-secretors, the *A* and *B* genes are active in the endodermal tissues and produce active transferases in the secretions, but these enzymes are unable to catalyse the synthesis of

A and B antigens in the secretions because their acceptor substrate, the H antigen, is absent.

The biochemically related Lewis system is described in Chapter 5.

H-deficient red cells

Phenotypes with H-deficient red cells are rare. Homozygosity for inactivating mutations in *FUT1*, the gene encoding the fucosyltransferase responsible for biosynthesis of H on red cells, results in red cells with no H antigen. As H-deficient red cells lack the precursor of A and B, they are always group O. If *A* or *B* genes are present, active A- or B-transferases will be present, but unable to produce A or B antigens in the absence of their acceptor substrate, the H antigen.

Red cell H-deficient individuals may be ABH secretors or non-secretors. Red cell H-deficient non-secretors (the Bombay phenotype) produce anti-H, plus anti-A and -B. Anti-H is clinically significant and has the potential to cause severe HTRs and HDFN. Consequently, anti-H can cause a serious transfusion problem because H-deficient phenotypes are rare and compatible blood is very difficult to find. Secretors with H-deficient red cells have H antigen in their secretions, but not on their red cells. They do not produce anti-H, but may make a related antibody called anti-HI, which is not usually active at 37°C and not generally considered clinically significant. Anti-HI is also quite a common antibody in individuals with A_1 phenotype.

Further complexities

There are many rare subgroups of A and B with different degrees of weakness of the A or B antigens. In some cases there is apparently normal secretion of A or B substance. The most commonly used names of A subgroup phenotypes are A_3, A_{end}, A_x, A_m, A_y, and A_{el}. They are defined by characteristic serological patterns and for most of the A subgroups one or more mutations in the *ABO* gene has been identified, but there is not always a straightforward correlation between genotype and phenotype.

Subgroups of B – B_3, B_x, B_m, and B_{el} – are serologically analogous to the subgroups of A. They are extremely rare.

On very rare occasions, the ABO groups appear to break the rules of Mendelian inheritance, with, for example, a group O parent of a child with a weak A phenotype (A_x). In one such family the father had the genotype A/O^1, with an *A* allele producing so little A antigen that it was not detectable by standard serological methods, but the child had the genotype A/O^2 in which the expression of the same *A* allele appears to have been enhanced by the O^2 allele in *trans*.

The phenotype called *cis*AB is very rare, but particularly interesting. Red cells with the *cis*AB phenotype are group AB, although both A and B are usually expressed somewhat weakly. The interesting point is that in *cis*AB both A and B are inherited from the same parent and can be passed on to the same child. The reason is that *cis*AB represents a single allele at the *ABO* locus that encodes a single transferase enzyme with dual A- and B-transferase activity. This *cis*AB-transferase has leucine at position 266, typical of A-transferase, but alanine at position 268, typical of B-transferase (compare with Fig. 3.4).

Acquired changes

On rare occasions group A people may acquire a B antigen and become group AB, although the B antigen is generally weak and there is some weakening of the A antigen. In most cases this phenomenon occurs in patients with diseases of the digestive tract, usually colon carcinoma. The usual explanation for acquired B is that bacterial enzymes in the blood remove the acetyl group from GalNAc, the immunodominant sugar of A antigen, to produce galactosamine, which is similar enough in structure to Gal, the immunodominant sugar of B antigen, to cross-react with some anti-B.

Weakening of A antigen is common in group A patients with acute myeloid leukaemia (AML). In some cases all red cells show weakness of the A antigen, whereas in others two populations of A and O red cells are apparent. Leukaemia-associated changes in B and H antigens are less common. Between 17% and 37% of patients with leukaemia have significantly lower A, B, or H antigenic expression compared with healthy controls. Occasionally, modifications of ABH antigens are manifested before diagnosis of malignancy and therefore indicate preleukaemic states. This leukaemia effect is probably epigenetic in origin, resulting from hypermethylation of the *ABO* promoter region.

A or B antigens on red cells can be abolished, *in vitro*, by converting them back to H antigen by removal of the immunodominant sugar with an appropriate enzyme, an exoglycosidase: α-N-acetylgalactosaminidase (A-zyme) or α-galactosidase (B-zyme). Highly efficient A-zymes and B-zymes have been produced from bacterial genes, with an aim of producing universal group O donor red cells from blood of all ABO groups.

Associations with disease and functional aspects

Some examples of associations between ABO group and disease have already been mentioned, notably HDFN, leukaemia, and bacterial-induced acquired B. Numerous other associations between ABO and diseases have been reported, mostly based on observed ABO phenotype frequency discrepancies between patients with the disease and the healthy population. For example, group A people appear to be more susceptible than those of other ABO groups to carcinoma of the stomach and colon. Group O individuals have a lower risk of thrombosis than those with A, B and AB phenotype. This probably arises from an effect on the presence of the A and B immunodominant sugars located on ADAMTS13, an enzyme responsible for clearance of the coagulation factor von Willebrand factor. It is likely that group O individuals are relatively resistant to severe malaria caused by *Plasmodium falciparum* infection.

Almost nothing is known about the functions of ABO antigens, on red cells or elsewhere in the body. ABH antigens are very abundant on red cells. The ABH antigens contribute to the glycocalyx or cell coat, an extracellular matrix of carbohydrate that protects the cell from mechanical damage and attack by pathogenic micro-organisms.

The Rh blood group system

CHAPTER 4

Introduction – Rh, not rhesus

The Rh blood group system was discovered in New York in 1939, with an antibody in the serum of a woman who had given birth to a stillborn baby and then developed a haemolytic reaction as the result of transfusion with blood from her husband. Levine and Stetson found that the antibody agglutinated the red cells of her husband and those of 80% of ABO compatible blood donors. Regrettably, Levine and Stetson did not name the antibody. In 1940, Landsteiner and Wiener made antibodies by injecting rhesus monkey red cells into rabbits. These antibodies not only agglutinated rhesus monkey red cells, but also red cells from 85% of white New Yorkers and appeared to be the same as Levine and Stetson's antibody and other human antibodies identified later. By 1962, however, it was clear that rabbit and guinea pig anti-rhesus reacted with a determinant that was genetically independent of that determined by the human antibodies, despite being serologically related. In consequence, the anti-rhesus antibodies were renamed anti-LW, after Landsteiner and Wiener, and the human antibodies remained as anti-D of the Rh (not rhesus) blood group system. LW is expressed more strongly on D+ than D− red cells, explaining the original error because weak antisera often fail to agglutinate D− red cells.

As early as 1943 Rh started to become complex. From their work with four other antisera, anti-C, -c, -E, and -e, detecting two pairs of antithetical antigens, Fisher and Race postulated three closely linked loci producing D or d, C or c, and E or e. Anti-d has never been found and does not exist. Wiener, in New York, worked with antibodies of the same specificities, but came up with a different genetical theory involving only one gene locus. In 1986, Tippett provided another alternative theory: two loci; one producing D or no D, the other producing C or c and E or e. Shortly after, Tippett's theory was validated by molecular genetic studies.

Essential Guide to Blood Groups, 2nd edition. By Geoff Daniels and Imelda Bromilow. Published 2010 by Blackwell Publishing Ltd.

Haplotypes, genotypes, and phenotypes

Although there are only two Rh gene loci, *RHD* and *RHCE*, the Fisher–Race theory of three loci, *D/d*, *C/c*, and *E/e*, is still appropriate for interpreting serological data because *C/c* and *E/e* represent different mutation sites within *RHCE*. No conclusive evidence of recombination between *D/d* and *C/c*, *C/c* and *E/e*, or *D/d* and *E/e* has been found.

The three pairs of alleles can comprise eight possible haplotypes. All have been identified and are shown in Table 4.1. These eight haplotypes can been paired to form 36 different genotypes. However, from these 36 genotypes, only 18 different phenotypes can be recognised by serological tests with anti-D, -C, -c, -E, and -e. This is because there is no anti-d, so homozygosity (*D/D*) and heterozygosity (*D/d*) for *D* cannot be distinguished serologically. For example, *DCe/dce* cannot be distinguished serologically from *DCe/Dce*. Furthermore, in *D/d* and *C/c* heterozygotes, it is not possible to determine whether *D* is in *cis* (on the same chromosome) with *C* or with *c*, so, for example, *DCe/dce* cannot be distinguished from *Dce/dCe*. The same applies to *D/d* and *E/e*, and to *C/c* and *E/e*; so by usual serological techniques *DcE/dce* cannot be distinguished from *Dce/dcE* and *DCe/DcE* cannot be distinguished from *DCE/Dce* (but see section on compound antigens).

The most common Rh phenotype in a Caucasian population is D+ C+ c+ E− e+. This is often written as DCe/dce (shorthand R_1r; Table 4.1). Although this is written in the format of a genotype, it is not a true genotype, but a probable genotype. It is not a true genotype because D+ C+ c+ E− e+ could also result from *DCe/Dce* (R_1R_0) or *Dce/dCe* (R_0r').

Table 4.1 Eight Rh haplotypes and their frequencies in English, Nigerian, and Hong Kong Chinese populations

Haplotype		Frequencies		
DCE	Shorthand	English	Nigerian	Chinese
DCe	R^1	42	6	73
dce	*r*	39	20	2
DcE	R^2	14	12	19
Dce	R^0	3	59	3
dcE	*r"*	1	Rare	Rare
dCe	*r'*	1	3	2
DCE	R^z	<1	Rare	<1
dCE	r^y	Rare	Rare	<1

It is a probable genotype because, in a Caucasian population, *DCe/dce* is 15 times more common than *DCe/Dce* and 650 times more common than *Dce/dCe*. In an African population, however, the haplotype *Dce* is more common than *dce*, so the probable genotype for D+ C+ c+ E– e+ would be *DCe/Dce*. The probable genotype for D+ C+ c+ E+ e+ is DCe/DcE (R_1R_2), but *DCe/dcE* (R_1r''), *DcE/dCe* (R_2r'), *DCE/dce* (R_zr), *Dce/DCE* (R_0R_z), and *Dce/dCE* (R_0r_y) are all alternatives of lower incidence. It is important to remember that probable genotypes and true genotypes are not always the same.

An alternative notation, with no genetical implications, is the numerical terminology of the International Society of Blood Transfusion (ISBT): D is RH1; C, RH2; E, RH3; c, RH4; and e, RH5. The common Rh phenotype D+ C+ c+ E– e+ is RH: 1,2,–3,4,5.

Biochemistry and molecular genetics

Rh phenotypes are controlled by two genes: *RHD*, which encodes the D antigen, and *RHCE*, which encodes the Cc and Ee antigens. Both genes have 10 exons and share about 94% sequence identity throughout all introns and exons. They are extremely unusual for closely linked homologous genes in that they are in opposite orientation on the chromosome; that is, in tail-to-tail configuration (5'*RHD*3'–3'*RHCE*5'), the coding strand of *RHD* becoming the non-coding strand of *RHCE*, and vice versa (Fig. 4.1). Another gene, *SMP1*, encoding a small membrane protein, is located between the Rh genes. *RHD* is flanked by two 9 kb regions of 98.6% identity, the *Rh boxes*.

RHD and *RHCE* encode proteins of 417 amino acids, although the N-terminal methionine is cleaved from the mature proteins. The RhD and RhCcEe proteins differ by between 31 and 35 amino acids, according to *RHCE* allele. Interpretation of the amino acid sequences predicts that the Rh proteins cross the membrane 12 times, providing six extracellular loops, the potential sites for expression of Rh antigens (Fig. 4.1). N- and C-termini are inside the cytosol. It is partly because the Rh proteins have this sort of polytopic structure that the Rh system is so complex. Rh antigens are very dependent on the shape of the molecule and may also involve interactions between more than one of the extracellular loops. Minor changes in the amino acid sequence, such as a single amino acid change, even within a membrane-spanning domain, can cause conformational changes that create new antigens and affect the expression of existing ones. Unlike most cell membrane proteins, the Rh proteins are not glycosylated.

Within the red cell membrane, the Rh proteins are associated with a glycoprotein called the Rh-associated glycoprotein (RhAG). RhAG shares

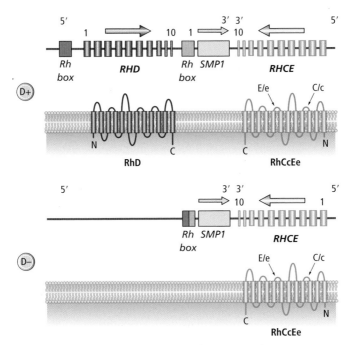

Fig. 4.1 Diagram representing the 10 exons of the *RHD* and *RHCE* genes in opposite orientation, the *Rh boxes* (regions of identity), and the *SMP1* gene. Below this are diagrammatic representations of Rh proteins, showing the N- and C-termini, the 12 membrane-spanning domains and the six extracellular loops. The C/c and E/e polymorphisms are determined primarily by amino acid substitutions on the second and fourth (from the N-terminus) extracellular loops of the RhCcEe protein. Above: D+ haplotype. Below: D− (deletion) haplotype.

33% identity with the Rh proteins and has a very similar arrangement in the membrane. Unlike the Rh proteins, RhAG is glycosylated, with a single *N*-linked sugar on the first extracellular loop, and it carries the antigens of the RHAG blood group system (Table 1.1). It is produced by the *RHAG* gene on chromosome 6. Although RhAG does not carry any Rh antigens, its presence is essential for expression of Rh antigens and in its absence no Rh antigens are expressed.

In addition, the membrane protein complex of Rh proteins and RhAG is part of the band 3/Rh ankyrin membrane protein macrocomplex, which also includes band 3 (AE1), glycophorins A and B, LW, and CD47. Evidence from studies on mice suggests that the Rh proteins are also part of the junctional protein complex, together with band 3, glycophorin C, Duffy, Kell, and Xk proteins (Fig. 4.2).

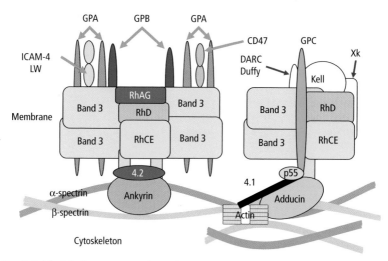

Fig. 4.2 Model of two proposed membrane complexes that include Rh proteins: (1) containing tetramers of band 3 and heterotrimers of RhD, RhCE, and RhAG, and linked to the spectrin matrix of the cytoskeleton through band 3, protein 4.2, and ankyrin; (2) containing band 3, RhD, and RhCE, and linked to the spectrin–actin junction through glycophorin C (GPC), p55, and protein 4.1 and though band 3 and adducin.

D antigen (RH1)

In the field of transfusion medicine, D is the most important Rh antigen, and the most important blood group antigen after A and B. Anti-D can cause severe and fatal haemolytic transfusion reactions (HTRs) and haemolytic disease of the fetus and newborn (HDFN). At least 30% of D− recipients of transfused D+ red cells make anti-D.

D+ and D− phenotypes are often referred to as Rh+ and Rh−. Between 82% and 88% of Europeans and North American Caucasians are D+; around 95% of black Africans are D+. D is a high frequency antigen in the Far East, reaching 100% in some populations.

D antigen expression varies quantitatively. Even among the common phenotypes there is readily detectable quantitative variation of D, with less D expressed in the presence of C (Table 4.2).

Molecular basis of the D polymorphism

The D− phenotype results from absence of the RhD protein. This explains why no antigen antithetical to D was found. Consequently, the symbol d simply represents an absence of D. In Caucasians, the D− phenotype almost always results from homozygosity for a deletion of *RHD* (Fig. 4.1).

Table 4.2 Estimated numbers of antigen sites per red cell (in thousands)

Phenotype	Antigens			
	D	C	c	e
DCe/dce	10–15	22–40	37–53	18–25
DCe/DCe	15–23	46–57	0	18–25
DcE/DcE	16–33	0	70–85	0
DCe/DcE	23–31	26–40	37–53	14–15
dce/dce	0	0	70–85	18–25

This deletion appears to have occurred between a 1463 bp region of identity in each of the *Rh boxes*. D+ people can be homozygous or hemizygous for the presence of *RHD*.

Sixty-six per cent of D– black Africans have an intact *RHD*, but this gene is inactive owing to a nonsense mutation in exon 6 (the codon for Tyr269 converted to a translation termination codon) and a 37 bp duplication in exon 4 that might introduce another premature termination codon. This inactive *RHD*, called *RHDΨ*, produces no D protein and no D antigen.

D variants

Numerous variants of D exist, mostly caused by mutations within the *RHD* gene. D variants have been ranked into two main classes:

1 **Weak D** (formerly D^u), in which the whole D antigen is expressed, but expressed weakly. Because all D epitopes are present, individuals with weak D cannot make anti-D when immunised by a normal, complete D antigen. Weak D is usually associated with amino acid substitutions in the membrane-spanning or cytosolic domains of the RhD protein, and are not exposed to the outside of the membrane.

2 **Partial D**, in which part of the D antigen is missing. That is, only some D epitopes are expressed, and these may be expressed normally or weakly. Because some or most of the D epitopes are missing, individuals with partial D can make an antibody to those epitopes they lack, following immunisation with complete D antigen, and this antibody behaves as anti-D in tests with red cells of common D phenotypes. Partial D is usually associated with amino acid changes in the exposed extracellular loops of the RhD protein.

However, this dichotomy is no longer valid. Some D variants have been classified as weak D (e.g. weak types 4.2 and 15), yet individuals with these variants have subsequently been found who have made anti-D. Some

Table 4.3 Some symbols given to D variants			
DII	DAR	DFR	DMH
DIIIa	DARE	DFW	DNAK
DIIIb	DAU	DHAR	DNB
DIIIc	DBA	DHK	DNU
DIVa	DBS	DHMI	DOL
DIVb	DBT	DHMII	DTO
DVa	DCC	DHO	DVL
DVI	DCS	DHR	DWI
DVII	DDE	DIM	DYU
	DEL	DIT	Weak D Type 1–73
	DFL	DLO	Weak D Type 1.1, 4.1, 4.2, 4.3

partial D antigens, such as DVI, have distinctly weakened expression of those epitopes they have. Consequently, the terminology is misleading and a new terminology is required. Table 4.3 provides a list of some of the symbols currently used to describe D variants.

Another type of D variant is DEL, in which the D is expressed so weakly it cannot be detected by conventional serological methods and requires specialist techniques, in particular adsorption and elution. Only about 3 in 1000 Japanese and Chinese are apparently D−, and a substantial proportion of those have the DEL phenotype. Despite the very low level of D expression on DEL red cells, they have still immunised D− patients to make anti-D following transfusion. Consequently, it is possible that all D variants have the potential to immunise D− transfusion recipients.

Numerous monoclonal antibodies to the D antigen have been produced. By definition, each monoclonal antibody detects only one epitope. Analyses of tests with many such antibodies against red cells expressing different D variant antigens has led to the definition of 30 reaction patterns, interpreted as 30 epitopes of D (epD).

Some D variant proteins express an antigen that is specific for that partial D antigen. For example, red cells with DIVa variant D always express Go^a (RH30), those with DV variant D express D^w (RH23), and those with DFR express FPTT (RH50).

Many D variants arise from missense mutations in *RHD*, which result in one or several amino acid substitutions in the RhD protein. In some cases, however, the mutation represents an exchange of genetic material between *RHD* and *RHCE*, so that sections of *RHD* are replaced by the equivalent section of *RHCE*. For example, in the most common type of DVI, exons 4, 5, and 6 of *RHD* are replaced by exons 4, 5, and 6 of *RHCE*, resulting in a hybrid protein in which part of the third extracellular loop

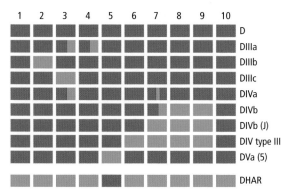

Fig. 4.3 Diagram of the 10 exons of nine examples of *RHD-CE-D* and one *RHCE-D-CE* (DHAR) genes responsible for D variant phenotypes. Red boxes, *RHD* exons; blue boxes, *RHCE* exons.

and the fourth and fifth loops have the sequence of a CcEe protein. Some examples are shown in Fig. 4.3.

Clinical significance of anti-D

Anti-D is clinically the most important red cell antibody in transfusion medicine after anti-A and -B. It has the potential to cause severe HTRs and D+ blood must never be given to a patient with anti-D. As at least 30% of D− recipients of transfused D+ red cells make anti-D, D+ red cells are not routinely transfused to D− patients.

Anti-D can cause severe HDFN. This occurs when IgG anti-D in an immunised mother crosses the placenta and facilitates destruction of D+ fetal red cells. The effects of HDFN caused by anti-D at its most severe are fetal death at about the seventeenth week of pregnancy. If the infant is born alive, the disease can result in hydrops and jaundice. If the jaundice leads to kernicterus, this usually results in infant death or permanent cerebral damage. In most cases of HDFN, the mother was immunised to produce anti-D by fetal D+ red cells during a previous pregnancy. These D+ red cells leak into the maternal circulation via a trans-placental haemorrhage, which generally occurs during delivery, but sometimes happens earlier in the pregnancy. Anti-D immunisation can be prevented, in most cases, by administration of a dose of anti-D immunoglobulin to the D− mother immediately after delivery of a D+ baby. It is still not absolutely clear how the anti-D immunoglobulin prevents immunisation, but it is probably because of rapid removal of the D+ fetal cells from the maternal circulation. In 1970, at the very beginning of the anti-D prophylaxis pro-gramme there were 1.2 deaths per thousand births in England and Wales due to HDFN caused by anti-D; by 1989 this figure had been reduced to 0.02. In order to prevent the less common occurrence of the mother being immunised during the course of the pregnancy, anti-D immunoglobulin may be administered to D+ pregnant women antenatally, and this has become the usual practice in many countries.

It is imperative that D+ red cells are never transfused to D− girls or pre-menopausal women. If a D− young woman is given D+ blood products, then anti-D immunoglobulin should be given.

Anti-D in women with a D variant antigen can cause severe HDFN in a fetus with a complete D antigen. If a woman known to have a D variant antigen gives birth to a D+ baby, she should be given anti-D immunoglobulin.

D testing

According to the UK guidelines, patient samples are tested in duplicate by direct agglutination with IgM monoclonal anti-D selected to give a negative result with category DVI cells. An antiglobulin test for detecting weak D variants should not be carried out. Patients with very weak D variants or DVI will be found to be D− and will receive D− blood. This will do no harm and will prevent the DVI patients from making anti-D and ensure that they receive anti-D immunoglobulin following a D+ pregnancy. For typing donors, however, at least one of the antibodies should detect DVI and weak forms of D. So DVI individuals are D+ donors but D− patients.

The prediction of D phenotype from fetal DNA is described in Chapter 7.

C, c, E, and e antigens (RH2, RH4, RH3, RH5)

C and c antigens are the products of alleles of *RHCE*. C and c have frequencies of 68% and 81%, respectively, in English blood donors. In black Africans the frequency of c is much higher and the frequency of C much lower, whereas in Eastern Asia the opposite is the case, C is higher and c lower (Table 4.4). E and e represent another pair of *RHCE* alleles. In all populations e is significantly more common than E (Table 4.4).

The numbers of C, c, and e antigen sites per cell is shown in Table 4.2.

Clinical significance of CcEe antibodies

All Rh antibodies should be considered to have the potential to cause HTRs and HDFN. For transfusion to a patient with an Rh antibody, antigen-negative blood should be provided wherever possible. Anti-c is clinically the most important Rh antigen after anti-D and often causes severe HDFN, whereas anti-C, -E, and -e rarely cause HDFN, and when they do the disease is generally (but not always) mild.

Table 4.4 Frequencies of C, c, E, and e antigens in three populations

Antigen	Population (%)		
	English	Nigerian	Chinese
C	68	17	94
c	81	99	43
E	29	23	36
e	98	99	96

Molecular basis of the C/c and E/e polymorphisms

The C/c and E/e polymorphisms are associated with amino acid substitutions in the RhCcEe protein. C/c primarily represents a Ser103Pro substitution in the second extracellular loop (Fig. 4.1), encoded by *RHCE* exon 2, although the situation is more complex than that. Ser103 is essential, but not sufficient, for C specificity: for full expression of C, the protein must have Ser103, Cys16, and some other downstream amino acids characteristic of the RhCcEe protein. Cys16 is not, however, a requirement for all epitopes of C as some rare Rh variants have Ser103, but Trp16 and express a weak, abnormal C. The c antigen is determined almost entirely by the presence of Pro103.

The E/e polymorphism is basically dependent on a Pro226Ala substitution, in the fourth extracellular loop, encoded by *RHCE* exon 5, although changes to other residues do have some effect on e expression.

Other Rh antigens

Of the 52 Rh antigens recognised by the ISBT, 20 have a frequency of between 1% and 99% in a least one major ethnic group, 21 are rare antigens, and 11 are antigens of very high frequency. Some of them are described briefly here.

Compound antigens: ce, Ce, CE, cE (RH6, RH7, RH22, RH27) and G (RH12)

Antibodies to compound antigens detect red cells when they have specific C or c and E or e antigens encoded by the same gene. For example, anti-ce (also known as anti-f) only reacts with cells of individuals who have a *dce* or *Dce* complex, that is, with c and e in *cis*. Consequently, red cells with the phenotype D+ C+ c+ E+ e+ will react with anti-ce, but not anti-Ce, if the genotype is *DCE/dce*, but will react with anti-Ce, but not anti-ce, if it is

DCe/DcE. Anti-ce is a common component of anti-c and anti-e sera, but is occasionally found as a single specificity. Most anti-C and anti-C+D sera contain some anti-Ce. Both anti-CE and anti-cE are rare antibodies.

Anti-G reacts with red cells that have D or C. That is, D+ C+, D+ C−, and D− C+ cells. The primary defining amino acid of C is Ser103 in the RhCcEe protein. The Rh D protein also has serine at this position. Consequently, anti-G recognises the presence of Ser103, whether it is in the context of a D protein or a CcEe protein, in contrast to anti-C, which is more conformationally dependent and only recognises the presence of Ser103 in the context of a CcEe protein. Anti-G is often present in sera containing anti-D plus anti-C, and can confuse serological investigations of HDFN.

C^w, C^x, MAR (RH8, RH9, RH51)

C^w is a relatively low frequency antigen in all populations, although its incidence is quite variable. In an English population C^w has a frequency of 2.6% and similar frequencies are found in most Caucasian populations. C^x is a rare antigen, with an incidence of between 0.1% and 0.3% in Caucasian populations. C^w and C^x are usually produced by *DCe* complexes that produce a weakened form of C. C^w is associated with a Glu41Arg substitution and C^x with an Ala36Thr substitution in a CcEe protein, with resultant conformational changes in the molecule responsible for the weakness of C. The high frequency antigen MAR is abolished by either the C^w or C^x substitution, so it appears that the presence of both Ala36 and Glu41 are required for MAR expression.

VS, V (RH20, RH10)

VS has a frequency of about 30–40% in black African populations, but is rare in other ethnic groups. VS is represented by a Leu245Val substitution in a CcEe protein and is associated with weak e. VS+ red cells are usually also V+, although about 20% of VS+ red cells lack V and, in addition to the Leu245Val substitution, have a Gly336Cys substitution. The haplotype containing the altered *RHCE* gene associated with a VS+ V− phenotype contains no *RHD*, but has an *RHD–CE–D* hybrid gene, which produces no D, but does produce an abnormal C.

Rh-deficient phenotypes – Rh_{null} and Rh_{mod}

A rare, but particularly interesting, Rh phenotype is Rh_{null}, in which the red cells express no Rh antigens. If immunised, Rh_{null} individuals can make anti-Rh29, an antibody to epitopes common to both Rh proteins, which reacts with all red cells apart from Rh_{null} cells.

Rh$_{null}$ has two types of inheritance:

1 Homozygosity for inactive Rh haplotypes. These individuals have no *RHD* (like most D− people) and are homozygous for *RHCE* containing an inactivating mutation, so that neither Rh protein can be produced.

2 Normal, active *RHD* and *RHCE* genes, but homozygosity for inactivating mutations in *RHAG*, an independent gene encoding the Rh-associated glycoprotein (RhAG), which is closely associated with the Rh proteins in the membrane. In the absence of RhAG, Rh antigens are not expressed. Some mutations in *RHAG* permit reduced quantities of RhAG to be produced, which results in low level expression of all Rh antigens: the Rh$_{mod}$ phenotype.

Rh$_{null}$ red cells are morphologically and functionally abnormal. Most Rh$_{null}$ and Rh$_{mod}$ individuals have some degree of haemolytic anaemia, which may be severe enough to merit splenectomy.

Putative function of the Rh proteins and RhAG

The Rh proteins and RhAG are homologous structures, with identical conformation in the membrane and 33% sequence identity. Their multiple membrane-spanning conformation with both termini in the cytosol (Fig. 4.1) is characteristic of membrane transporters. RhAG and, to a lesser extent, the Rh proteins have amino acid sequence homology with proteins involved in ammonia transport in lower organisms. Yeast cells lacking ammonium transporters fail to grow in low ammonium medium, but will grow successfully in that medium following transfection with *RHAG*. Transport of an ammonium analogue into *Xenopus* oocytes was enhanced 8- to 10-fold following transfection of the cells with *RHAG*, transient expression of RhAG in a human cell line (HeLa) enhanced the permeability for ammonium ions and for ammonia, and red cells of *Rhag* knockout mice have severely impaired ammonia transport. The RhAG and Rh protein complex in red cells could be involved in ammonium transport; with red cells carrying ammonium away from the brain, to the liver or kidney for metabolism or excretion.

Two of the primary functions of the red cell are transport of oxygen and conversion of carbon dioxide to bicarbonate, by carbonic anhydrase in the red cell cytoplasm. Rh$_{null}$ red cell have substantially reduced CO_2 membrane permeability and the macrocomplex involving RhAG and band 3 could function as a gas exchange channel for carbon dioxide and possibly oxygen. The macrocomplex is ideally located to channel CO_2 to and from carbonic anhydrase and O_2 to and from haemoglobin.

Other blood groups

ABO and Rh are the most clinically significant and best known of the blood group systems, yet there are 28 other systems of diverse clinical and biological relevance (see Table 1.1). These systems are described in this chapter. In addition, there are other antigens, which have not been allotted to a system, most of which are either of very high or very low frequency.

The Kell system

The antigen often referred to as Kell, but correctly named K or KEL1, is the original antigen of the Kell system and the first blood group antigen to be identified following the discovery of the antiglobulin test in 1946. The Kell system now consists of 32 antigens numbered from KEL1 to KEL35, with 3 obsolete. Some pairs and one triplet of Kell antithetical antigens are listed in Table 5.1.

Kell glycoprotein and the *KEL* gene

The Kell system antigens are located on a red cell membrane glycoprotein that is N-glycosylated, but not O-glycosylated (see Chapter 1). It spans the membrane once and is unusual because its short N-terminal domain is in the cytosol and its large C-terminal domain is outside the membrane (see Fig. 1.1). The extracellular domain has five or six N-glycosylation sites and 15 cysteine residues, and is extensively folded by disulphide bonding. Kell system antigens are sensitive to disulphide bond reducing agents such as dithiothreitol (DTT) and 2-aminoethylisothiouronium bromide (AET).

The Kell protein has structural and sequence homology with a family of zinc-dependent endopeptidases that process a variety of peptide hormones. Although the function of the Kell glycoprotein is not known,

Essential Guide to Blood Groups, 2nd edition. By Geoff Daniels and Imelda Bromilow. Published 2010 by Blackwell Publishing Ltd.

Table 5.1 Antithetical antigens of the Kell blood group system

Relative frequency				Molecular basis	Polymorphic in:
High		**Low**			
k	KEL2	K	KEL1	Thr193Met	Caucasians, Africans
Kp^b	KEL4	Kp^a	KEL3	Arg281Trp	Caucasians
		Kp^c	KEL21	Arg281Gln	Not polymorphic
Js^b	KEL7	Js^a	KEL6	Leu597Pro	Africans
K11	KEL11	K17	KEL17	Val302Ala	Not polymorphic
K14	KEL14	K24	KEL24	Arg180Pro	Not polymorphic
Not identified		VLAN	KEL25	Arg248Gln	Not polymorphic
		VONG	KEL28	Arg248Trp	

it is enzymatically active and is able to cleave the biologically inactive peptide big endothelin-3 to create the biologically active vasoconstrictor endothelin-3.

The *KEL* gene is located on chromosome 7. It is organised into 19 exons of coding sequence.

Kell system antigens

K (KEL1) has a frequency of about 9% in Northern Europeans, about 1.5% in people of African origin, and is rare in East Asia. The k (KEL2) antigen is antithetical to K and is of high frequency in all populations. K and k result from a single nucleotide polymorphism (SNP) in exon 6, which encodes Met193 in K and Thr193 in k. As N-glycosylation at Asn191 is dependent on the presence of Thr193, the k-active Kell glycoprotein is N-glycosylated at Asn191, whereas the K-active molecule is not.

Kp^a (KEL3) is found in about 2% of Caucasians and is not present in Africans or in Japanese. An antithetical antigen, Kp^b (KEL4), is of high frequency in all populations. Whereas 2.3% of Caucasians are Kp(a+), only 1.2% of K+ Caucasians are Kp(a+). Nine per cent of Caucasians are K+, but only 2.7% of Kp(a+) people from the same population are K+. This strong allelic association was confirmed by family studies. Only one example of the *KKp^a* haplotype has been found. Kp^c (KEL21), an antigen of very low frequency, is the product of a another allele of *Kp^a* and *Kp^b*. *KEL* alleles encoding the three Kp antigens differ by single base substitutions within codon 281 (exon 8): *Kp^a*, TGG, Trp281; *Kp^b*, CGG, Arg281; *Kp^c*, CAG, Gln281.

Js^a (KEL6) is almost completely confined to people of African origin. The frequency of Js^a in African Americans is about 16%. Js^b (KEL7) is of high frequency in all populations. Js^a represents Pro597; Js^b, Leu597.

Some other Kell antigens are shown in Table 5.1. In addition, presence of the low frequency antigens Ul^a, K23, and KYO, and absence of the high frequency antigens K12, K13, K18, K19, K22, TOU, RAZ, KALT, KTIM, KUCI, KASH, KANT, and KELP all result from single amino acid substitutions in the Kell glycoprotein.

Kell system antibodies

Antibodies of the Kell system should be considered potentially clinically significant, both from the point of view of causing severe haemolytic disease of the fetus and newborn (HDFN) and haemolytic transfusion reactions (HTRs). Patients with Kell system antibodies should be transfused with antigen-negative blood whenever possible. Kell system antibodies are usually immunoglobulin G (IgG) and predominantly IgG1.

HDFN caused by anti-K differs from that resulting from anti-D. Anti-K HDFN is associated with lower concentrations of amniotic fluid bilirubin than anti-D HDFN of comparable severity. Postnatal hyperbilirubinaemia is not prominent in babies with anaemia caused by anti-K. There is also reduced reticulocytosis and erythroblastosis in the anti-K disease, compared with anti-D HDFN. The Kell glycoprotein appears on erythroid progenitors at a much earlier stage of erythropoiesis than Rh antigens. Consequently, anti-K probably facilitates phagocytosis by macrophages in the fetal liver of K+ erythroid progenitors at an early stage of development, before they produce haemoglobin.

Anti-K is the most common immune red cell antibody outside of the ABO and Rh systems: one-third of all non-Rh red cell immune antibodies are anti-K. K– girls and women of child-bearing age should be transfused with K– blood. Some anti-K directly agglutinate K+ red cells, but an antiglobulin test is the method of choice for detection.

K$_o$ phenotype

Like most blood group systems, Kell has a null phenotype (K$_o$) in which none of the Kell system antigens are expressed. K$_o$ individuals may produce anti-Ku (anti-KEL5) if immunised, an antibody that reacts with all cells except those of the K$_o$ phenotype. Homozygosity for a variety of nonsense mutations, missense mutations, and splice site mutations have been associated with K$_o$ phenotype.

McLeod syndrome, McLeod phenotype, and Kx (XK1) antigen

McLeod syndrome, which is associated with acanthocytosis and a variety of muscular and neurological defects, is very rare, X-linked, and found almost exclusively in boys. It results from hemizygosity for inactivating mutations and deletions of the *XK* gene, causing absence of Xk protein, which expresses Kx (the only antigen of the Kx system). Xk protein is linked to the Kell glycoprotein through a single disulphide bond. McLeod syndrome is associated with McLeod phenotype, in which Kell system antigens are expressed weakly and Km (KEL20) as well as Kx are absent.

Deletion of part of the X chromosome that includes *XK* may also include the gene responsible for X-linked chronic granulomatous disease (CGD). When transfused, CGD patients with McLeod syndrome usually produce anti-Kx plus anti-Km, making it almost impossible to find compatible donors. It is recommended, therefore, that transfusion of boys with CGD and McLeod syndrome should be avoided if possible.

The Duffy system

The antigens of the Duffy system reside on a glycoprotein encoded by the Duffy gene (*FY* or *DARC*), which consists of two exons, exon 1 encoding only the first seven amino acids of the Duffy glycoprotein.

Fyᵃ (FY1) and Fyᵇ (FY2)

In Caucasians and Asians the Duffy polymorphism consists of two antigens, Fyᵃ and Fyᵇ, giving rise to three phenotypes, Fy(a+b−), Fy(a+b+), and Fy(a−b+) (Table 5.2). The *Fyᵃ* and *Fyᵇ* alleles represent an SNP in exon 2 of the *FY* gene, encoding Gly42 and Asp42, respectively.

In Africans there is a third allele, called *Fy*, more common than *Fyᵃ* and *Fyᵇ*. *Fy* produces no Duffy glycoprotein on red cells, and hence neither Fyᵃ nor Fyᵇ, nor any other Duffy antigen. Individuals homozygous for *Fy* have the red cell phenotype Fy(a−b−), the frequency of which varies from about 70% in African Americans to 100% in the Gambia (Table 5.2).

The coding region for the *Fy* allele in Africans is identical to that of the *Fyᵇ* allele, encoding Asp42. *Fy* produces no Duffy glycoprotein or Fyᵇ antigen in red cells because of a mutation in the promoter region of the *FY*

Table 5.2 Duffy phenotypes and genotypes in three populations

Phenotype	Genotype		Frequencies (%)		
	Caucasian & Asian	African	Europeans	Africans	Japanese
Fy(a+b−)	*Fyᵃ/Fyᵃ*	*Fyᵃ/Fyᵃ* or *Fyᵃ/Fy*	20	10	81
Fy(a+b+)	*Fyᵃ/Fyᵇ*	*Fyᵃ/Fyᵇ*	48	3	15
Fy(a−b+)	*Fyᵇ/Fyᵇ*	*Fyᵇ/Fyᵇ* or *Fyᵇ/Fy*	32	20	4
Fy(a−b−)		*Fy/Fy*	0	67	0

gene. This mutation prevents binding of the erythroid-specific GATA-1 transcription factor and prevents expression of the gene in erythroid tissue. Fy(a–b–) Africans lack Duffy glycoprotein from their red cells, but not from other tissues. This explains why they do not make anti-Fy^b and only very rarely make anti-Fy3 (see below).

Fy^a and Fy^b are very sensitive to most proteolytic enzymes, including papain, ficin, and bromelin, but are not destroyed by trypsin. A weak form of Fy^b is called Fy^x.

Anti-Fy^a and -Fy^b

Anti-Fy^a is a relatively common antibody, whereas anti-Fy^b is rare. IgG1 usually predominates, generally detected by an antiglobulin test. Naturally occurring examples are very rare.

Anti-Fy^a and -Fy^b may cause immediate or delayed HTRs. Although generally mild, some have proved fatal. These antibodies have also been responsible for HDFN, varying from mild to severe.

Fy3 and Fy5

Very rare non-Africans with Fy(a–b–) red cells are homozygous for inactivating mutations in their *FY* genes. These individuals would not be expected to have Duffy glycoprotein on their red cells or in any other tissues. All were found through the presence of anti-Fy3 in their sera. Fy3 is present on all cells except those of the Fy(a–b–) phenotype. Unlike Fy^a and Fy^b, Fy3 is protease resistant.

Like Fy3, Fy5 is absent from cells of the Fy(a–b–) phenotype, but, unlike Fy3, Fy5 is also absent from cells of the Rh$_{null}$ phenotype. The reason for this association between Duffy and Rh is not known. Anti-Fy5 has only been found in multiply transfused black people. Anti-Fy3 has been responsible for immediate and delayed HTRs and anti-Fy5 for delayed HTRs.

The Duffy glycoprotein, a receptor for chemokines

The Duffy glycoprotein, also known as the Duffy antigen receptor for chemokines (DARC), is a red cell receptor for a variety of chemokines including interleukin 8 (IL-8) and melanoma growth stimulatory activity (MGSA). It traverses the membrane seven times, with a 63 amino acid, extracellular, N-terminal domain containing two potential N-glycosylation sites, and a cytoplasmic C-terminal domain (Fig. 5.1). This arrangement is characteristic of the G-protein-coupled superfamily of receptors, which includes chemokine receptors.

Duffy and malaria

The Duffy glycoprotein is a receptor for *Plasmodium vivax* merozoites, the parasite responsible for a form of malaria widely distributed in Africa,

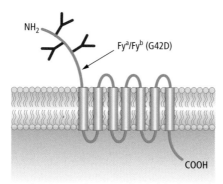

Fig. 5.1 The Duffy glycoprotein (DARC), with a glycosylated external N-terminal domain, seven membrane-spanning domains, and cytoplasmic C-terminus.

but less severe than malaria resulting from *P. falciparum* infection. Red cells with the Fy(a–b–) phenotype are resistant to invasion by *P. vivax* merozoites. Consequently, the *Fy* allele confers a selective advantage in areas where *P. vivax* is endemic and this probably balances with any disadvantage resulting from absence of the chemokine receptor on red cells.

The Kidd system

Jkᵃ (JK1) and Jkᵇ (JK2); anti-Jkᵃ and -Jkᵇ

Jkᵃ and Jkᵇ are the products of alleles, with similar frequencies in most populations (Table 5.3). Jkᵃ represents aspartic acid and Jkᵇ asparagine at position 280 in the Kidd glycoprotein.

Kidd antibodies are dangerous as they may cause severe immediate HTRs. They are also a very common cause of delayed HTRs, probably because they are often not detected, owing to their tendency to drop to low or undetectable levels in the plasma. Anti-Jkᵃ and -Jkᵇ only very rarely cause severe HDFN.

Anti-Jkᵃ and -Jkᵇ often bind complement. They are usually IgG or IgG plus IgM.

Table 5.3 Frequencies of Jkᵃ and Jkᵇ antigens in three populations

Antigen	Frequencies (%)		
	Europeans	Africans	Asians
Jkᵃ	76	92	73
Jkᵇ	72	49	76

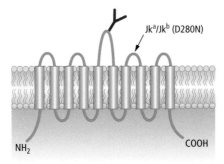

Jk^a/Jk^b (D280N)

NH$_2$

COOH

Fig. 5.2 The Kidd glycoprotein, a urea transporter, with cytoplasmic N- and C-terminal domains, 10 membrane-spanning domains, and an N-glycan on the third extracellular loop.

Jk(a−b−) and Jk3

The null phenotype, Jk(a−b−) Jk:−3, usually results from homozygosity for a silent gene at the *JK* locus. Although very rare in most populations, Kidd null is relatively common in Polynesians with a frequency of around 1 in 400. The Polynesian null allele contains a splice site mutation in intron 5 resulting in the loss of exon 6 from the mRNA. Immunised individuals with the Jk(a−b−) phenotype may produce anti-Jk3, which can cause immediate or delayed HTRs.

The Kidd glycoprotein is a urea transporter

The Kidd antigens are located on a red cell urea transporter, with 10 potential membrane-spanning domains, cytoplasmic N- and C-termini, and one extracellular N-glycosylation site (Fig. 5.2). When red cells approach the renal medulla, which contains a high concentration of urea, the urea transporter permits rapid uptake of urea and prevents the cells shrinking in the hypertonic environment. As the red cells leave the renal medulla, urea is transported rapidly out of the cells, avoiding swelling of the cells and preventing the red cells carrying urea away from the kidney.

Unlike normal red cells, Jk(a−b−) cells are not lysed by 2*M* urea, and this may be used as a method for screening for Jk(a−b−).

The MNS system

MNS is a highly complex blood group system consisting of 46 antigens. Like Rh, much of the complexity arises from recombination between closely linked homologous genes, *GYPA* and *GYPB*, which encode the glycoproteins glycophorin A (GPA) and glycophorin B (GPB).

M (MNS1) and N (MNS2); anti-M and -N

M and N (as determined by most anti-N reagents) are antithetical antigens and polymorphic in all populations tested. Frequencies of the common phenotypes in Caucasians are M+ N– 28%, M+ N+ 50%, and M– N+ 22%. Anti-M is a relatively common 'naturally occurring' antibody, whereas anti-N is quite rare. Most anti-M and -N are not active at 37°C and are not clinically significant. They can generally be ignored in transfusion practice and, if room temperature incubation is eliminated from compatibility testing and screening for antibodies, they will not be detected. When M or N antibodies active at 37°C are encountered, IAT-compatible blood should be provided. Very occasionally anti-M and -N have been implicated as the cause of immediate and delayed HTRs and anti-M has, very rarely, been responsible for severe HDFN.

M and N are located at the N-terminus of GPA, a red cell glycoprotein that crosses the membrane once and has a highly glycosylated, sialic acid-rich, extracellular domain. M-active GPA has serine at position 1 and glycine at position 5; N-active GPA has leucine at position 1 and glutamic acid at position 5. GPA is very abundant, with about 10^6 copies per red cell.

S (MNS3) and s (MNS4); anti-S and -s

S and s are another pair of antithetical antigens of the MNS system. Phenotype frequencies in Caucasians are as follows: S+ s– 11%, S+ s+ 44%, and S– s+ 45%. Family studies showed tight linkage between M/N and S/s. Anti-S and -s are generally IgG antibodies active at 37°C. They have been implicated in HTRs and have caused severe and fatal HDFN.

S and s represent a Met29Thr polymorphism in GPB, a glycoprotein resembling GPA. The amino terminal 26 amino acids of GPB are usually identical to those of the N form of GPA. Consequently, in almost all Caucasians and most people of other races GPB expresses 'N'. GPB is much less abundant than GPA, with only about 20,000 copies per cell, and most anti-N do not detect the 'N' antigen on GPB.

S– s– U– phenotype and anti-U

Red cells of about 1% of African Americans and a higher incidence of black Africans are S– s– and lack the high frequency antigen U (MNS5). If immunised, these individuals may produce anti-U. Anti-U has been responsible for severe and fatal HTRs and HDFN.

The S– s– U– phenotype can result from homozygosity for a deletion of the coding region of *GYPB*, the gene encoding GPB. Other, more complex molecular phenomena involving hybrid genes may also give rise to a S– s– phenotype, with expression of a variant U antigen.

Other MNS antigens and antibodies

The other MNS antigens are either of high or low frequency in most populations. The similarity of sequence between certain regions of *GYPA* and *GYPB* may occasionally lead to *GYPA* pairing with *GYPB* during meiosis. If recombination then occurs, either by crossing-over or by a less well-defined mechanism called gene conversion, then a hybrid gene can be formed consisting partly of *GYPA* and partly of *GYPB*. A large variety of these rare hybrid genes exist and give rise to low frequency antigens and, in the homozygous state, to phenotypes that lack high frequency antigens. Red cells of some of these phenotypes react with an antibody called anti-Mi^a (MNS7) and were grouped together as the Miltenberger series, but this classification is now obsolete.

Mur antigen (MNS10) is rare in Caucasians and Africans, but has a frequency of about 7% in Chinese and 10% in Thais. Anti-Mur has the potential to cause severe HTRs and HDFN. In Hong Kong and Taiwan, anti-Mur has been found to be the most common blood group antibody other than anti-A and -B. It is important that in South East Asia red cell panels used for screening patient sera for antibodies contain Mur+ cells.

The Diego system

Band 3, the red cell anion exchanger

The 22 antigens of the Diego system are located on band 3, the common name for the red cell anion exchanger, AE1. Band 3 is a major red cell membrane glycoprotein with approximately 10^6 copies per red cell. It has a long cytoplasmic N-terminal domain, a transmembrane domain that traverses the membrane 14 times, and a cytoplasmic short C-terminal domain (Fig. 5.3). There is a single N-glycan on the fourth extracellular loop. Band 3 has at least two functions: the rapid exchange of HCO_3^- and Cl^- ions, important in CO_2 transport, and attachment of the red cell membrane to the cytoskeleton. Tetramers of band 3 form the core of the band 3–Rh ankyrin macrocomplex of red cell membrane proteins and band 3 is also a component of the proposed junctional complex (see Fig. 4.2). The band 3 gene (*SLC4A1*) consists of 20 exons of coding sequence and is on chromosome 17.

Di^a (DI1) and Di^b (DI2); anti-Di^a and -Di^b

Di^a, the original Diego antigen, is very rare in people of European and African origin, but has a frequency of 5% in Chinese and Japanese and a higher frequency in the native peoples of North and South America, reaching 54% in the Kainganges Indians of Brazil. Di^b is a high frequency antigen in almost all populations. Di^a and Di^b represent an amino acid

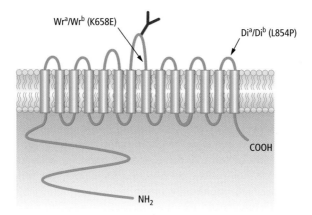

Fig. 5.3 Band 3, the Diego glycoprotein and anion exchanger, with cytoplasmic N- and C-terminal domains, 14 membrane-spanning domains, and an N-glycan on the fourth extracellular loop.

substitution in the seventh extracellular loop of band 3: Leu854 in Di^a and Pro854 in Di^b.

Anti-Di^a and -Di^b are usually IgG1 plus IgG3 and generally require an antiglobulin test for detection, although a few directly agglutinating examples have been found. Anti-Di^a occasionally bind complement and lyse untreated red cells. Anti-Di^a, which is present in 3.6% of multitransfused patients in Brazil, can cause severe HDFN. Anti-Di^b has, very rarely, been responsible for serious HDFN.

Wr^a (DI3) and Wr^b (DI4); anti-Wr^a and -Wr^b

The low frequency antigen Wr^a and its antithetical antigen of extremely high frequency, Wr^b, represent an amino acid substitution in the fourth loop of band 3: Lys658 in Wr^a and Glu658 in Wr^b. Despite homozygosity for the Glu658 codon in the band 3 gene, Wr^b is not expressed in the rare phenotypes where the MN glycoprotein, GPA, is absent or where that part of GPA close to insertion into the red cell membrane is absent. This provides strong evidence for an interaction between band 3 and GPA within the red cell membrane.

Anti-Wr^a is a relatively common antibody, usually detected by an antiglobulin test, but sometimes by direct agglutination of red cells. Anti-Wr^a are mostly IgG1, but sometimes IgM or IgM plus IgG. Anti-Wr^a has been responsible for severe HDFN and for HTRs. Alloanti-Wr^b is rare and little is known about its clinical significance, but autoanti-Wr^b is a relatively common autoantibody and may be implicated in autoimmune haemolytic anaemia.

Other Diego system antigens

In the last few years, 17 antigens, all of very low frequency, have been shown to represent amino acid substitutions in band 3 and have joined the Diego system.

The Lewis system

Lewis antigens are carbohydrate structures carried on glycolipids. Unlike most other blood group antigens, they are not produced by erythroid cells, but become incorporated into the red cell membrane from the plasma. There are two main antigens of the Lewis system, Le^a (LE1) and Le^b (LE2), but they are not the products of alleles. The product of the Lewis gene, *FUT3*, is a fucosyltransferase that catalyses the transfer of fucose from GDP-fucose to the Type 1 precursor of H to form Le^a and to Type 1 H to form Le^b (Fig. 5.4, and see Figs 3.2 and 3.3). There are four Lewis phenotypes (Table 5.4).

1 **Le(a+b−).** Only found in ABH-non-secretors. Owing to the inactivity of the *FUT2* encoded fucosyltransferase, which is characteristic of non-secretors (see Chapter 3), only Type 1 H precursor and not Type 1 H is present in secretions, so only Le^a is made and incorporated into the red cell membrane.

2 **Le(a−b+).** Only found in ABH-secretors. Most Type 1 H precursor is converted to Type 1 H in secretions by the *FUT2* encoded fucosyltransferase,

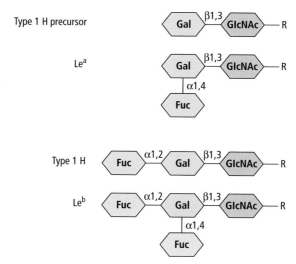

Fig. 5.4 Diagrammatic representation of Le^a and its precursor, Type I H precursor, and Le^b and its precursor, Type 1 H. R, remainder of molecule.

Table 5.4 Phenotypes and genotypes of the Lewis system

Phenotype	Genotype		Approximate frequency (%)		
	Lewis (*FUT3*)	Secretor (*FUT2*)	Caucasians	African Americans	Chinese
Le(a+b–)	*Le/Le* or *Le/le*	*se/se*	22	20	0
Le(a–b+)	*Le/Le* or *Le/le*	*Se/Se* or *Se/se*	72	55	62
Le(a+b+)	*Le/Le* or *Le/le*	*Se^w/Se^w* or *Se^w/se*	0	0	27
Le(a–b–)	*le/le*	Any	6	25	11

Le and *Se*, active alleles; *le* and *se*, inactive alleles; *Se^w*, weakly active allele.

so predominantly Le^b, and very little Le^a, is formed and only Le^b is detected on the red cells.

3 **Le(a+b+).** Only found in ABH-secretors with a weak secretor (*FUT2*) gene. Less Type 1 H precursor is converted to Type 1 H than in Le(a–b+), so both Le^a and Le^b are abundant in secretions and are detected on the red cells.

4 **Le(a–b–).** Regardless of ABH-secretor type, Le(a–b–) red cells have no Lewis antigens owing to homozygosity for inactivating mutations in the Lewis (*FUT3*) gene and no production of Lewis transferase or Lewis antigens.

The Lewis antigens ALe^b (LE5) and BLe^b (LE6) result from the conversion of Type 1 A and B structures by the Lewis transferase, in A-secretors and B-secretors, respectively.

Lewis antibodies, which are only made by individuals with Le(a–b–) red cells, are not generally considered clinically significant, as they are seldom active at 37°C.

Some other blood group systems

P1PK

P1 has a frequency of about 80% in Caucasians. It is an oligosaccharide antigen located on a glycolipid of the paragloboside series. Most anti-P1 do not agglutinate red cells at 25°C and are not considered clinically significant. The other antigen of this system is P^K.

Lutheran

Lutheran is a complex system comprising 20 antigens, including four antithetical pairs: Lu^a/Lu^b (His77Arg); Lu6/Lu9 (Ser275Phe); Lu8/Lu14

(Met204Lys); and Au^a/Au^b (Thr529Ala). The Lutheran glycoprotein is an adhesion molecule of the immunoglobulin superfamily that binds the extracellular matrix glycoprotein laminin. The extremely rare Lu_{null} phenotype arises from homozygosity for inactive *LU* genes. Heterozygosity for inactivating mutations in the erythroid transcription factor, EKLF, is responsible for In(Lu), an Lu_{mod} phenotype with extremely weak expression of Lutheran antigens and also weakened expression of several other blood group antigens including P1, In^b, and AnWj. Hemizygosity for a mutation in the gene for the major erythroid transcription factor, GATA-1, resulted in an Lu_{mod} phenotype with an X-linked mode of inheritance. Lutheran antibodies are not generally considered clinically significant.

Yt

Yt^a and Yt^b (His353Asn) are antithetical antigens on acetylcholinesterase. Yt antibodies are not generally considered clinically significant.

Xg

Xg^a is encoded by *XG*, an X-linked gene, and has a frequency of about 66% in males and 89% in females. Anti-Xg^a is not clinically significant.

Scianna

Scianna consists of seven antigens on the adhesion molecule ERMAP, all of very high or very low frequency. No Scianna antibody has been incriminated in an HTR or in severe HDFN.

Dombrock

The Dombrock system consists of seven antigens: the polymorphic antithetical antigens Do^a and Do^b (Asn265Asp), and the high frequency antigens Gy^a, Hy, Jo^a, DOYA, and DOMR. Anti-Gy^a is the antibody characteristically produced by immunised individuals with the Dombrock-null phenotype. Anti-Do^a and -Do^b have been responsible for HTRs. The Dombrock glycoprotein has a structure characteristic of an ADP-ribosyltransferase.

Colton

Co^a (Ala45) is a high frequency antigen; Co^b (Val45) its antithetical antigen with an incidence of about 8% in Caucasians, but lower in other ethnic groups. Anti-Co3 reacts with all red cells except those of the extremely rare Colton-null phenotype. Colton antibodies have been implicated in severe HDFN and in HTRs. The Colton antigens are located on aquaporin-1, a water channel.

Landsteiner–Wiener (LW)

LW^a and LW^b (Gln70Arg) are antithetical antigens of high and low frequency, respectively. Anti-LW^{ab} reacts with all red cells except those of the extremely rare LW-null phenotype and Rh_{null} cells, which are also LW(a–b–). LW antibodies are not generally considered clinically significant. The LW glycoprotein is intercellular adhesion molecule-4 (ICAM-4), an adhesion molecule of the immunoglobulin superfamily, and is a component of the band 3–Rh ankyrin macrocomplex (see Fig. 4.2).

Chido/Rodgers
The nine antigens of the Chido/Rodgers systems are not true blood group antibodies as they are not produced by erythroid cells. They are located on the fourth component of complement (C4), which binds to the red cells from the plasma.

Gerbich
The six Gerbich antigens of very high frequency and five antigens of very low frequency are located on the sialoglycoproteins glycophorin C (GPC) or glycophorin D (GPD), or on both. The two glycoproteins of different size arise from initiation of translation at two different sites on *GYPC* mRNA. They are part of the proposed junctional complex of membrane proteins (see Fig. 4.2) and are important in functioning as a link between the membrane and the cytoskeleton. Anti-Ge3 has caused HDFN.

Cromer
The 13 high frequency and three low frequency Cromer antigens are located on the complement-regulatory glycoprotein, decay accelerating factor (DAF or CD55). Cromer antibodies are not usually clinically significant.

Knops
The nine antigens of the Knops system are located on the complement-regulatory glycoprotein, complement receptor-1 (CR1 or CD35). Knops system antibodies are not clinically significant.

Indian
The low frequency antigen In^a (Arg46) and its antithetical antigen In^b (Pro46), plus two other high frequency antigens, are located on CD44, a ubiquitous molecule with multifarious functions that binds the extracellular matrix glycoprotein hyaluronan. Indian antibodies are not generally considered clinically significant.

I
I, the sole antigen of this system, represents branched carbohydrate chains that are internal structures of the ABH-active oligosaccharides. The product of the I gene (*GCNT2*) is an enzyme (β1,6-*N*-acetylglucosaminyl-transferase), which catalyses the branching of straight carbohydrate

(*N*-acetylactosamine) chains. The straight chains express i antigen. Red cells of newborn infants are I–, but express i strongly. Branching of the oligosaccharide chains results in weakening of i and expression of I, which reaches maximum strength between 6 and 18 months of age. Very rare individuals, who are homozygous for inactivating mutations in *GCNT2*, never convert i to I, and have the adult i phenotype and usually produce alloanti-I. These antibodies are generally IgM and are only rarely active at 37°C. In Eastern Asia adult i phenotype is usually associated with congenital cataracts, but this is not the case in Caucasians. This is because mutations in Asian adult i are in *GCNT2* mRNA transcripts that are expressed in haemopoietic tissues and in epithelial tissues that are responsible for normal function of the lens, whereas the Caucasian mutations are in transcripts that are only expressed in haemopoietic tissues.

Potent I autoantibodies may be haemolytic and cause cold haemagglutinin disease (CHAD). Antibodies with i specificity are autoantibodies and are often found in patients with infectious mononucleosis.

Antigens that do not belong to a blood group system

In addition to those belonging to the 30 blood group systems, there are many antigens that have not been shown to belong to a system. These are mostly antigens of either very high or very low frequency.

Antibodies to high frequency antigens are a transfusion hazard as compatible blood is often very difficult to obtain. Anti-Vel, -Lan, and -AnWj have caused severe HTRs. Anti-Vel are particularly dangerous antibodies, as they are usually IgM and complement-activating, and cause severe immediate HTRs. Anti-MAM has caused severe HDFN.

There are 18 authenticated antigens with frequencies well below 1%, which have not been shown to belong to a blood group system. Most antibodies to these antigens do not appear to be clinically significant, but anti-JFV, -Kg, -JONES, -HJK, and -REIT have all been responsible for HDFN.

Bg is the name given to human leucocyte antigen (HLA) Class I antigens expressed on mature red cells: Bg^a represents HLA-B7; Bg^b, HLA-B17; and Bg^c, HLA-A28 (cross-reacting with HLA-A2). Many individuals, however, do not express Bg antigens on their red cells, despite having the corresponding HLA antigens on their lymphocytes. Although there are a few reports of Bg antibodies causing HTRs, they are mostly only significant as contaminants in reagents.

Clinical significance of blood group antibodies

In immunohaematology, antibodies may be classified as 'naturally occurring' or 'immune'. This means that antibody molecules may be present in an individual regardless of the fact that there has been no known stimulus such as the transfusion of antigen different blood or feto-maternal haemorrhage. Both 'naturally occurring' and 'immune' antibodies can be of importance in immunohaematology. Antibodies can be further divided into categories 'alloantibody', raised in response to an antigen lacking on the cells of the individual, or 'autoantibody', which has specificity against an antigen present on the individual's own red cells.

Most human antibodies with which we are familiar are polyclonal in origin, being of broader specificity than monoclonal antibodies, which can have single epitope specificity. These antibodies can be of importance in certain clinical situations such as the ones described briefly below.

1 Haemolytic transfusion reaction (HTR), when an antibody destroys antigen-positive transfused red cells. The most severe HTRs are generally caused by antibodies to antigens of the ABO system, which are immunoglobulin M (IgM) in nature and initiate the complement cascade through to the membrane attack complex (MAC) (Fig. 6.1 and see Fig. 2.1), causing lysis of cells intravascularly. Other antibodies, IgG in nature, generally either do not initiate complement activation or only up to the C3 stage and red cells are cleared extravascularly.

2 Haemolytic disease of the fetus and newborn (HDFN), when an IgG maternally derived antibody, which is directed against a paternally derived antigen present on the fetal/neonatal red cells, crosses the placenta and destroys the cells.

3 Haemolytic anaemia (HA), when an autoantibody directed against 'self' antigens is produced and causes increased red cell destruction. These antibodies may be non-specific or may possess a defined specificity,

Essential Guide to Blood Groups, 2nd edition. By Geoff Daniels and Imelda Bromilow. Published 2010 by Blackwell Publishing Ltd.

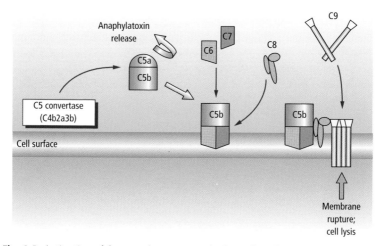

Fig. 6.1 Activation of the complement cascade through to the membrane attack complex (MAC), producing 'pores' in the red cell, allowing solutes to enter and escape, resulting in cell lysis (and see Fig. 2.1).

often against a high incidence antigen. The antibodies may be warm reactive or react optimally in the cold.

Antibody production and structure

Antibodies are immunoglobulins secreted by the progeny of B lymphocytes that differentiate in response to antigen stimulation. Multiple clones of B cells produce polyclonal antibodies with molecular heterogeneity whereas monoclonal antibodies are biochemically identical being produced by a single B-cell clone (Figs 6.2 and 6.3).

All antibody molecules are similar in overall structure, having a common core arrangement of two identical light chains, either κ (kappa) or λ (lambda), and two identical heavy chains, which denote the isotype of the antibody. In humans the different isotypes are IgA, IgD, IgE, IgG, and IgM (Table 6.1).

The genes for antibody production are located on chromosome 14 band q32 for the heavy chains, and chromosome 2p11 and 22q11 for κ and λ light chains, respectively. Each chain is separately synthesised before the antibody molecule is assembled. Figure 6.4 depicts the basic form of IgG possessing two gamma heavy chains and either κ or λ light chains. The antibody binding site is made up from the variable regions of the heavy and light chains.

IgM antibodies are in the form of a pentamer (Fig. 6.4).

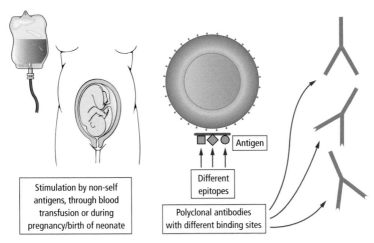

Fig. 6.2 Schematic diagram showing the production of polyclonal antibodies of human origin.

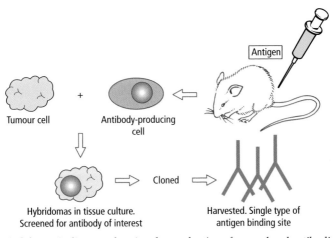

Fig. 6.3 Schematic diagram showing the production of monoclonal antibodies.

IgG molecules are flexible and sub-classes have different properties and effector functions; for example, the longer hinge region of IgG3 contributes to the flexibility of the molecule, it is more efficient at complement activation, and less molecules per cell are required to initiate red cell destruction processes (Table 6.2).

Table 6.1 Properties of immunoglobulins

Antibody isotype	Subclass	Heavy chain	Serum conc. (mg/mL)	Half-life (days)	Complement fixation
IgA	IgA1	alpha α	3	6	Not classical +/0 Alternative
	IgA2	alpha α	0.5	6	
IgD	None	delta δ	Trace	3	0
IgE	None	epsilon ε	Trace	2.5	
IgG	IgG1	gamma γ	9	23	++
	IgG2	gamma γ	3	23	+
	IgG3	gamma γ	1	23	+++
	IgG4	gamma γ	0.5	23	0
IgM	None	mu μ	1.5	5	++++

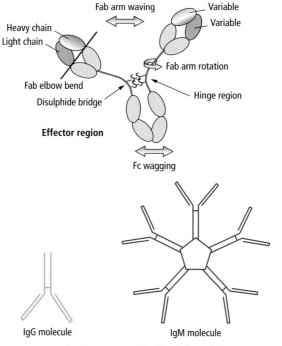

Binding site: 2 per IgG molecule; variable regions of heavy (γ) and light (κ or λ chains)

Fab arm waving

Heavy chain
Light chain

Variable
Variable

Fab arm rotation

Fab elbow bend
Disulphide bridge

Hinge region

Effector region

Fc wagging

IgG molecule   IgM molecule

Fig. 6.4 Representation of IgG indicating the flexibility of the molecule and line drawings of IgG and IgM showing the pentamer structure of IgM with 10 binding sites, composed of variable regions of heavy (μ) chains and κ or λ light chains.

Table 6.2 Some properties associated with the subclasses of IgG

	IgG1	IgG2	IgG3	IgG4
Amino acids in hinge region	16	12	62	>16
	Flexible	Restricted	Greater flexibility	Intermediate IgG1 and IgG2
Enzymes	Intermediate	Resistant	Susceptible	Intermediate

Factors affecting the clinical significance of antibodies

All antibodies exert their biological effects by binding to the appropriate antigens. An antibody is said to be clinically significant when it has the potential to initiate accelerated destruction of red cells carrying the appropriate antigen. Thus, alloantibodies, whether naturally occurring or of immune origin, and autoantibodies can be of clinical importance. Several factors have a role:

1 specificity of the antibody;
2 concentration and avidity of the antibody;
3 thermal amplitude (below 30°C unimportant);
4 immunoglobulin class/sub-class of antibody;
5 activity of the mononuclear phagocytic system;
6 antigen site density and mobility of the antigen in the membrane;
7 volume of red cells administered; and
8 soluble blood group substances (may neutralise the antibody, e.g. Lewis substance).

Antibody specificity

Antibody screening should be undertaken as part of all pre-transfusion testing and is also an integral part of antenatal testing. As a minimum, screening should be performed using at least two non-pooled test cells covering all important antigens, with certain critical antigens present in double-dose as recommended by local and/or national guidelines. Screening should use as a minimum the indirect antiglobulin test (IAT) to detect antibodies of potential clinical importance that may provoke a transfusion reaction or cause HDFN (Fig. 6.5). If an antibody known to be implicated in transfusion reactions is identified, then antigen-negative blood must be selected for cross-matching. (Fig. 6.6).

The antibody specificity is probably the single most helpful indication as to whether a particular alloantibody may be capable of promoting

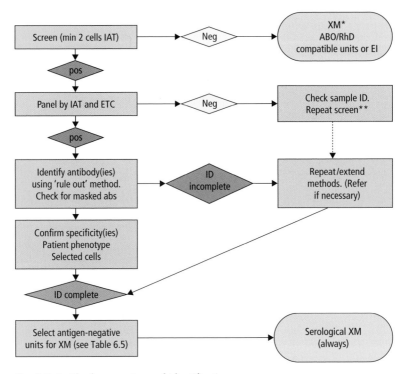

Fig. 6.5 Antibody screening and identification.
* Serological cross-match by IAT or electronic cross-match and issue if extended screen performed and validated computer system in place. It is essential to correctly select and check the ABO group of units for transfusion.
** May need to select a new/different batch of cells. Rule out contamination and/or technical error. If reproducible, check for low frequency antigen/antibody reaction and identify causative antibody (may need to refer).

accelerated red cell destruction. In conjunction with its optimal thermal range, it may be possible to predict its clinical significance. Antibodies that do not react below 37°C are generally not considered to be able to initiate significant red cell destruction, although antibodies within the ABO system should always be considered of potential importance (Table 6.3).

Haemolytic transfusion reactions (HTR)

HTRs may result from intravascular or extravascular destruction of red cells and may be acute (immediate) or delayed (up to 14 days post-transfusion).

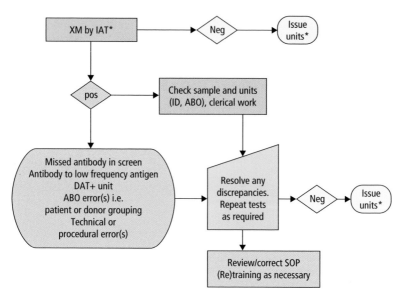

Fig. 6.6 Serological cross-matching (XM).
*It is essential to correctly select and check the ABO group of units for transfusion. XM by IAT at 37°C detects IgG antibodies of potential importance. ABO antibodies may not be detected. The 'immediate spin' technique (5 minutes' incubation at room temperature (20–25°C)) may be used to help ensure ABO compatibility.

Table 6.3 Selected blood group antibodies and their clinical importance

Clinically important	Important only when reactive at 37°C	Sometimes significant	Clinically benign
ABO	Le^a	Yt^a	Knops
Rh	M, N	Ge	Chido/Rodgers
Kell	P$_1$	Gy^a	Xg^a
Duffy	Lutheran	Hy	Bg
Kidd	A$_1$	Sd^a	Cs^a
Ss			Yk^a, McC^a
Vel			JMH

Intravascular red cell destruction

Intravascular red cell destruction presents as haemoglobinuria and haemoglobinaemia due to the ultimate haemolysis of the transfused cells. IgM anti-A and -B are most often implicated. Lewis antibodies only very

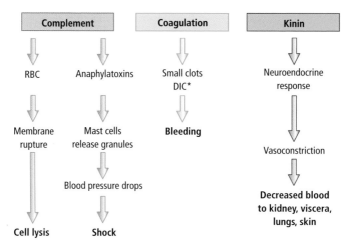

Fig. 6.7 Biological systems involved in an acute haemolytic transfusion reaction (HTR) and the potential consequences. *DIC-disseminated intravascular coagulation.

rarely cause intravascular haemolysis. During complement activation, C3a and C5a anaphylatoxins are released (Figs 2.1 and 6.1) and are responsible for many of the signs and symptoms of an acute HTR. C5a is a far more potent mediator of inflammation than C3a, which accounts for the more serious problems associated with transfusion reactions due to intravascular destruction initiated by an IgM antibody (Fig. 6.7).

Extravascular red cell destruction

Extravascular red cell destruction is usually associated with IgG antibodies, which fail to activate complement or fix complement only up to the C3 stage of the cascade. Red cells coated with IgG1 and/or IgG3 adhere at the hinge region of the antibody molecule to Fc receptors on macrophages and are phagocytosed or destroyed by a cytotoxic mechanism. Phagocytosis is favoured when there is moderate coating of the red cells. If the antibody does not fix complement, such as virtually all IgG anti-D and some IgG anti-K, -S and -Fy^a, the cells are mainly destroyed in the spleen, where conditions of haemoconcentration occur. Free IgG in the circulation prevents significant destruction at other sites because the circulating IgG molecules compete for the binding sites on macrophages. When complement components are also present on the red cells, a synergistic relationship between the two occurs and the cells are destroyed even more effectively. This generally takes place in the liver where there are abundant phagocytic cells possessing receptors for both IgG and the C3c component of complement. Antibodies against antigenic determinants in the Kidd blood group system are often described as 'complement dependent'. Recent evidence suggests that only IgM, and not IgG, Kidd antibodies are able to bind complement. Initially, destruction of cells sensitised with complement due to activation by IgM or IgG antibody is rapid but slows abruptly because the C3b becomes inactivated and quickly cleaved to C3dg. Macrophages do not have receptors for IgM or C3dg.

Cells heavily coated with IgG1 and/or IgG3 antibodies usually trigger destruction by the antibody dependent cytotoxicity mechanism. Lysosomal enzymes released by mononuclear cells effect the destruction; however, both phagocytosis and cytotoxic mechanisms can occur at the same time.

Haemolytic disease of the fetus and newborn (HDFN)

The cornerstone of antenatal care is regular testing for antibodies of potential importance and monitoring the alloimmunised pregnancy accordingly (Fig. 6.8).

IgM antibodies, while efficient at provoking complement activation and so are responsible for most cases of transfusion-related intravascular red cell destruction, do not cross the placenta and are therefore not implicated in the fetal red cell destruction associated with HDFN. The most severe manifestation of HDFN is caused by IgG antibodies directed against D, c, or K antigens on the fetal red cells, but any IgG antibody has the potential to cause the disease with varying severity.

Fetal cells sensitised by IgG1 and/or IgG3 antibody are destroyed with the release of breakdown products of haemoglobin that can be measured in the amniotic fluid. Amniocentesis to assess fetal well-being is less accurate earlier in the gestation period than after about 24 weeks' gestation.

More accurate data can be obtained from fetal blood sampling to measure the haemoglobin (Hb) and haematocrit (HCT) directly. In severe HDFN, intrauterine transfusions (IUT) may be required to maintain the pregnancy when the fetal HCT falls to <0.25 at 18–26 weeks or 0.3 after 26 weeks, the aim being to bring the HCT to around 0.35–0.40.

Non-invasive methods to assess fetal anaemia include ultrasound scanning and measurement of middle cerebral artery (MCA) Doppler velocity. An anaemic fetus has enhanced cardiac output and a decreased blood viscosity, leading to increased blood flow velocity that can be used as a screening tool to assess anaemia.

In vitro tests for assessing the ability of the antibody to initiate destruction of sensitised red cells are useful laboratory tools, such as antibody dependent cell-mediated cytotoxicity (ADCC). This measures the release

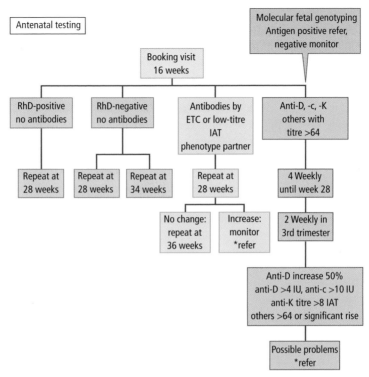

Fig. 6.8 Recommended schedule for antenatal testing in non-alloimmunised and alloimmunised pregnancies based on UK guidelines. ETC, enzyme treated cells; IAT, indirect antiglobulin test.

of Cr^{51} as an indication of target red cells lysed by lymphocytes or monocytes used in the assay as effector cells. The chemiluminescence test (CLT) measures adherence and phagocytosis of sensitised red cells by effector cells in the presence of luminol. The CLT results are expressed as a percentage of the monocyte response to positive control cells and results over 30% are consistent with moderate to severe disease. Titres of antibodies implicated in HDFN are not predictive of the outcome of the pregnancy, but serve as a guide to the level of antibody at any given stage of the pregnancy. Quantification of levels of anti-D and -c can indicate the need for treatment of the fetus. Generally, if the anti-D is >4 IU/mL or increases by 50% in comparison with a previous result, or if the anti-c is >10 IU/mL, the fetus may require treatment. Anti-D levels of >15 IU/mL are associated with severe HDFN.

There is no method for quantification of anti-K and even an antibody with a low titre can cause severe HDFN. Anti-K causes HDFN by affecting early red cell precursors, before haemoglobin production. Therefore, in HDFN due to anti-K there is little destruction of circulating mature red cells making measurement of breakdown products of haemoglobin in the amniotic fluid less informative.

HDFN due to anti-D has been reduced since the introduction of prophylactic anti-D administration and routine antenatal anti-D administration reduces the incidence even further. The incidence of RhD sensitisation has been reduced to about 11 cases per 10,000 births with severe disease in less than 1 per 20,000 births. Anti-K is found in around 1/1000 pregnant women but only about 1/20,000 pregnancies are affected with HDFN.

Interventions in alloimmunised pregnancies can prevent serious morbidity and mortality (Table 6.4). These interventions are necessary to prevent and/or treat severe fetal anaemia, which can lead to congestive heart failure, intrauterine growth retardation, and hydrops due to hepatic dysfunction. *In utero*, bilirubin released from the breakdown of haemoglobin is partly cleared by the placenta and so it may not be until the infant is born that serious problems develop, when exchange transfusion may be indicated.

Exchange transfusion removes about 90% of the neonate's antigen-positive cells, which may only survive 2–3 days in the most severe HDFN. It also removes up to 50% of the available intravascular bilirubin and reduces circulating maternal antibody. If these measures are not taken, there is a risk of kernicterus, when the bilirubin crosses the blood–brain barrier and permeates the basal ganglia, resulting in high morbidity and mortality in affected infants.

Cross-matching for infants under 4 months old

- Determine maternal and infant's ABO/D types (forward grouping only on infant's red cells, preferably ×2).
- Screen maternal serum for the presence of irregular antibodies (use infant's serum if maternal blood unavailable).
- Direct antiglobulin test (DAT) on infant's red cells.
- If there is no evidence of irregular, clinically important antibodies and the infant's cells are DAT negative, then blood of the same ABO/Rh type may be administered, without a cross-match, even for repeat transfusions, ensuring that the donor unit has been correctly typed.
- If an antibody is present, donor blood should be cross-matched using the maternal sample. Infants of group O mothers can be given group O red cells, to avoid complications due to passive IgG anti-A/B.
- If the DAT is positive, then the cause should be established using the appropriate laboratory tests on maternal and infant's samples.

Table 6.4 Some recommendations for the transfusion of an affected fetus or neonate

	HCT*/Hb†/bilirubin	Treatment	Remarks	Transfusion requirements
Prenatal	HCT <0.25 at 18–26 weeks' gestation (0.3 after 26 weeks' gestation)	Serial IUT (2–3 weekly, depending on results)	Aim to raise HCT to 0.45 Volume: desired HCT – fetal HCT × feto-placental blood volume, ÷ unit HCT – desired HCT	O (low titre haemolysin) or ABO identical. RhD and K negative (DCe/DCe for anti-c). <5 days: HCT 0.75; CMV negative, irradiated (25 Gy minimum)
Postnatal	Bilirubin >100 μmol/L and rapidly rising with cord Hb <8 g/dL	Exchange transfusion	Hb 13.6 g/dL lower limit of normal in term infants Double-volume (total): 160–200 mL/kg, depending on clinical condition	HCT 0.5–0.6. D and K negative, compatible with maternal serum. <5 days old: CMV negative, irradiated. Screened for HbS where appropriate

CMV, cytomegalovirus.

* HCT: the haematocrit is the relative volume of blood occupied by the red cells. Normal values are between 0.35 and 0.52. Lowered HCT values are associated with anaemia, bone marrow failure, and numerous other pathogenic conditions.

† Hb: haemoglobin is the oxygen transport metalloproteins in red cells. Normal level in full-term neonates is between 13.6 (lower limit) and 19.6 g/dL. Low Hb is associated with anaemia, destruction of red cells, dyserythropoeisis, and many other pathogenic conditions.

Autoantibodies

In autoimmune haemolytic anaemia (AIHA) autoantibody reacts with all normal red cells, including the patient's own. The autoantibody is most often IgG in nature. In cold antibody haemolytic anaemia, the autoantibody tends to be IgM and can activate complement. The peripheral blood sample generally shows the presence of C3d on the red cells. Paroxysmal cold haemoglobinuria (PCH) is most often associated with post-viral infection in children. The antibody is a biphasic haemolysin, IgG in nature, and with P specificity. Atypical haemolytic anaemias (HA) are known to occur; for example, combining warm and cold antibody involvement and HA in which the direct antiglobulin test is negative. Some drug-induced HAs are clinically indistinct from warm antibody immune haemolytic anaemia (WAIHA).

In addition to autoantibodies, there may also be alloantibodies present that can cause destruction of transfused red cells. It is therefore very important to determine if an alloantibody of clinical importance is present. This can be achieved by adsorption of the autoantibody to reveal any underlying specific antibody. Antigen-negative blood must be selected for transfusion in these cases. Determining the specificity of the auto-antibody, for example by elution from the DAT positive cells, is generally of little help in HA.

Tests to assess the potential significance of an antibody

When an antibody is of questionable importance or is directed against an antigen of high frequency, it may be necessary to establish the likelihood of red cell destruction in the event of transfusion or pregnancy. During an alloimmunised pregnancy, tests to demonstrate the relative strength and/or concentration of an antibody include quantification and/or titration end point estimation. Quantification of anti-D and -c are possible by an autoanalyser technique, in parallel with standard antibodies of known concentration in IU/mL or by flow cytometry. It must be noted that titre end points and/or scores do not correlate with the outcome of alloimmunised pregnancies. Other tests, which are based upon the *in vivo* destruction mechanisms, include the monocyte monolayer assay (MMA), and the chemiluminescence test (CLT) which measure monocyte phagocytosis, and the antibody dependent cell-mediated cytotoxicity (ADCC).

These methods can also be used to assess the biofunctional activity of an antibody in the plasma of a potential transfusion recipient, when compatible blood is impossible to find; for example, to distinguish antibodies capable of causing the increased destruction of transfused incompatible red cells from antibodies that are clinically benign. These assays are useful if a patient has an antibody to a high incidence antigen or an antibody whose specificity has not been identified and blood transfusion is necessary. If a patient has a mixture of antibodies that cause problems in obtaining donor blood negative for all target antigens, these tests can indicate which antibodies need to be considered of primary importance in terms of preventing a transfusion reaction.

An *in vivo* method for demonstrating the clinical significance of an antibody is to tag a small aliquot (0.5–1.0 mL) of donor red cells with Cr^{51}. The radioactivity is then measured after 3 (base line), 10, and 60 minutes after injection, in order to provide a measure of risk should the complete unit be transfused. This test is rarely performed now, not least because the results obtained from a small aliquot of tagged cells do not necessarily reflect the outcome of transfusion of a large amount of red cells.

Decision-making for transfusion

When an antibody has been detected and identified as potentially significant, and the patient requires a blood transfusion, Table 6.5 indicates an approach to transfusion therapy. The table is not exhaustive and other antibodies may be encountered for which a decision must be made according to the clinical situation and the results of tests. Where multiple antibodies exist, the specificities known to be of potential importance need to be considered and blood that is antigen negative for all such antibodies should be administered. Consideration may be given to autologous donation or testing of family members to find compatible blood, or it may be necessary to contact a Rare Donor Registry such as at the International Blood Group Reference Laboratory, Bristol, UK.

Patients who are likely to require long-term transfusion therapy can be fully phenotyped for the major blood group systems so that closely matched blood can be selected. When a patient has been recently transfused, so that serological phenotyping is not possible, the blood group genotype of the patient can be determined by molecular methods (see Chapter 7).

Closely matched blood can prevent immunisation to important antigens and lessens the subsequent burden of supplying compatible blood for patients who develop multiple antibodies. Not all workers agree with this approach, however, as not all patients will be responders to antigenic stimuli. The benefits must therefore be weighed against the costs of phenotyping both patients and donors.

As a final note, blood should only be transfused when it will benefit the patient. The best transfusion is no transfusion!

Table 6.5 Choice of blood for transfusion of patients with antibodies

Antigen-negative donor red cells	Anti-A, -B, -A,B Anti-M (at 37°C), -S, -s, -U All Rh antibodies (not -Cw) Anti-Lu^b, -Lu3 All Kell antibodies (not Kp^a, -Ul^a, K17) All Duffy and Kidd antibodies Anti-Di^a, -Di^b, Wr^b Anti-Sc1, -Co^a, -H (in O$_h$), -Kx, -I (allo at 37°C), -P, -PP1Pk, -Vel, -AnWj	–
Serologically compatible by IAT at 37°C	Anti-A1, -N, -En^a, -low frequency MNS antigens, -C^w, -P1, -Lu^a, -Kp^a, -Ul^a, -K17, -Le^a, -Le^b, -Le^{a+b}, -Wr^a, -Yt^b, -Xg^a, -Do^a, -Do^b, -Co^b, -HI, -In^a, Autoanti-I	When the antibodies are demonstrated by IAT at 37°C
Ideally antigen negative	Anti-Sc3, -Co3	Antigen negative blood extremely rare. 'Least incompatible' may be required to be transfused, with extra caution where the physician deems transfusion necessary
Serologically 'least incompatible'	Chido/Rodgers, Gerbich, Cromer, Knops, JMH, -Er^a, -LKE, -Sd^a	
	Anti-LW^a, -LW^{ab}	D– cells, unless with anti-c in DCe/DCe patient
	Antibodies to other high frequency Lu antigens Anti-Gy^a, -Hy, -Jo^a, -Yt^a, -Lan, -At^a, -Jr^a	Antigen-negative cells for strong antibodies

When assessing an antibody, the points reviewed here are meant as a general guide. Each antibody must be assessed as being unique to the situation. Reports in the literature have shown that antibodies generally considered unimportant, can, under certain circumstances, be rendered significant and vice versa.

Blood grouping from DNA

Almost all the genes for human blood groups have now been cloned and the molecular bases for all of the clinically important blood group polymorphisms determined. Consequently, it is now possible to predict a person's blood group phenotype from their DNA with a high degree of accuracy. Some applications of this technology and the methods applied are described in this chapter.

Fetal blood grouping

Currently, a common application is predicting the RhD group of the fetus of a pregnant woman with a blood group antibody, to assist in assessing the risk of haemolytic disease of the newborn (HDFN). If the fetus is D+, then the pregnancy should be closely monitored; if it is D−, unnecessary intervention can be avoided.

Prior to 2001 the usual source of fetal DNA was amniocytes or cells of the chorionic villi, obtained by amniocentesis or chorionic villus sampling. Both of these procedures are invasive and associated with increased risks of spontaneous abortion. In addition, there is a 20% risk of transplacental haemorrhage with amniocentesis, which could boost the maternal antibody, enhancing the risk of severe HDFN.

Cell-free fetal DNA derived from the placenta is detectable in the blood of pregnant women. The quantity of this fetal DNA, which cannot be separated from maternal DNA, increases throughout the pregnancy, finally achieving about 10% of total cell-free DNA in the plasma. Fetal D type can be predicted reliably from the fetal DNA in the plasma of D− pregnant women from the beginning of the second trimester, avoiding invasive procedures. Almost all laboratories applying this technology

Essential Guide to Blood Groups, 2nd edition. By Geoff Daniels and Imelda Bromilow. Published 2010 by Blackwell Publishing Ltd.

for diagnostic purposes employ real time quantitative polymerase chain reaction (PCR) with Taqman chemistry.

Most D– Caucasians are homozygous for a deletion of *RHD* (see Chapter 4), so most molecular tests for D typing involve amplifying one or more regions of *RHD* to determine whether the gene is present. Variant *RHD* genes introduce complications. For example, in *RHDΨ*, which is relatively common in Africans, all exons of *RHD* are present, but no D antigen is expressed on the red cells. In other variants, such as *RHDVI*, parts of *RHD* may be replaced by the equivalent region of *RHCE*, yet a variant D antigen is present on the red cells. False predictions caused by these variants can be reduced by taking them into account in the design of the test. A problem in all tests on fetal DNA in maternal plasma arises from the large quantity of maternal DNA present in the DNA preparation, complicating the inclusion of satisfactory internal controls to test for successful amplification of fetal DNA.

Tests on free fetal DNA in maternal plasma for predicting fetal K of the Kell system and Rh C, c, and E are also applied as a routine diagnostic service by a few laboratories.

It is practice in many countries to offer one or two doses of anti-D immunoglobulin antenatally, usually at around 28–34 weeks' gestation, to prevent D immunisation during the pregnancy. As the D phenotype of the fetus is not known, this therapy is offered to all pregnant D– women, yet about 40% in a Caucasian population will be carrying a D– fetus and receive the treatment unnecessarily. Trials of high-throughput methods have demonstrated that accurate fetal D testing in all D– pregnant women is feasible and will be standard practice within the next few years, at least in some European countries, avoiding unnecessary treatment of pregnant women with blood products.

Blood group typing of patients and donors

Most blood group polymorphisms of clinical significance, other than those of the ABO and Rh systems, result from single nucleotide polymorphisms (SNPs), which can be detected by a rapidly growing variety of technologies, many of which are available commercially. Conventional methods, involving the use of restriction enzymes or allele-specific primers, are being replaced by technologies with a potential for higher throughput, such as those involving microarrays (Fig. 7.1) or coloured microbeads, in which numerous SNPs can be analysed in a single test. Complications can arise from null phenotypes, which usually result from inactivating mutations within the gene, meaning that no antigen is produced despite apparently being encoded. These null phenotypes are

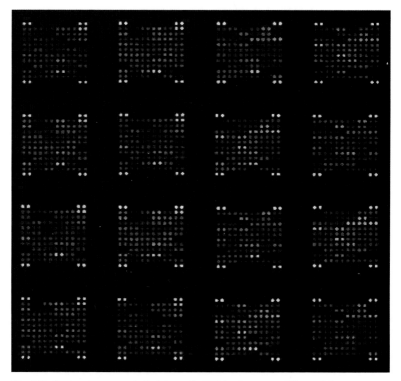

Fig. 7.1 Computer generated picture of a DNA microarray (BloodChip, Progenika), with the red spots representing positive results and the green spots negative results.

very rare, but they should be taken into account in any populations where they reach a significant frequency.

It is difficult to determine blood group phenotypes by conventional serological methods on red cell samples from patients who have recently received multiple blood transfusions. Transfusion-dependent patients, such as those with haemoglobinopathies, often benefit from determination of their blood group phenotypes, either to assist in identification of their blood group antibodies or to provide matched blood so that they do not make multiple antibodies. When DNA is prepared from blood from transfused patients, PCR-based tests will reveal the blood group genotype of the patient and not that of the donors, probably because of the low numbers of nucleated cells transfused.

Molecular testing is of particular value when red cells give a positive direct antiglobulin test, making serological testing difficult. This usually applies to patients with autoimmune haemolytic anaemia as a full predicted phenotype provides clues to which clinically significant allo-antibodies might be masked by the presence of an autoantibody.

Molecular tests can be used for testing patients and donors when serological reagents are of poor quality or in short supply. For example, anti-Do^a and -Do^b can be haemolytic, yet satisfactory serological reagents for antigen testing are not available. Some Rh variants are relatively common in people of African origin, but are difficult to define serologically. Molecular tests can be employed to assist in finding suitable blood for sickle cell disease patients.

Numerous variants of D exist: some result in loss of D epitopes and some in reduced expression of D; most probably involve both (see Chapter 4). In many cases D variants cannot be distinguished by serological methods, so molecular methods are required for their identification.

DEL is a rare D phenotype in which the D antigen is undetectable by routine serological methods, but, as DEL is associated with the presence of a mutated *RHD* gene, it can easily be detected by molecular methods. Transfusion of DEL red cells might be capable of immunising a D– recipient to make anti-D and in a few regions of Europe all apparent D– donors are screened for *RHD*, which would also catch other forms of very weak D expression. This practice is not considered necessary by most transfusion services.

The application of high-throughput testing for multiple blood group SNPs makes it practical to type numerous blood donors for most clinically significant polymorphisms in order to establish a large database of fully typed donors. Such a database would be very useful for providing blood for transfusion-dependent patients, such as sickle cell disease patients or patients with other haemoglobinopathies. A SNP detection method has been applied for the routine detection of blood group and platelet antigen polymorphisms on more than 10,000 donors in Quebec, Canada.

Molecular methods are already starting to replace serological methods for some blood group typing, and this trend will continue. However, it is unlikely that molecular methods will replace routine serological ABO typing in the foreseeable future. Compared with DNA tests, serological tests are quick, easy to perform, relatively cheap, and highly accurate, whereas the molecular genetics of ABO is very complex with numerous variants.

Quality assurance in immunohaematology

Quality can be defined as a 'degree of excellence' and assurance as 'positive assertion'. Quality assurance (QA) of a process therefore means that confidence in the outcome can be guaranteed at a pre-defined level of quality. In transfusion, this is of prime importance and the ideal to be achieved is zero defects throughout the transfusion chain.

Total quality management (TQM) in laboratory procedures and processes stresses the importance of collecting data as a basis for decision making and problem solving. In this way, the whole transfusion process can be analysed and improved in the long term.

Total quality is not the responsibility of one person or one department; quality is everybody's business and the only way to minimise risks and avoid potential errors is for all individuals to take responsibility for their actions.

Achieving total quality

1 Set appropriate standards.
2 Ensure good communication.
3 Full documentation and document control. Traceability of all laboratory procedures, including quality control (QC) results, batch numbers, expiry dates of reagents, and staff identification.
4 Training, in-house, relevant and continuous.
5 Standard operating procedures (SOPs), which must be complied with.
6 QC for individual procedures, which must reflect the technology used and be appropriate.
7 External assessment by participating in QA schemes to monitor standards, spot trends, help to reduce errors.
8 Establish an internal incident reporting and investigation system.

Essential Guide to Blood Groups, 2nd edition. By Geoff Daniels and Imelda Bromilow. Published 2010 by Blackwell Publishing Ltd.

Frequency and specificity of control material

Controls must be carried out for all test procedures; generally, at least daily and when new batches of reagents are introduced. Single tests, for example in an emergency situation, require that controls are included at the same time. Tables 8.1 and 8.2 present an overview of controls for

Table 8.1 Selection of material for quality control of routine laboratory procedures

Test protocol	Material (minimum)	Frequency (minimum)	Remarks
ABO forward typing	A1 and B cells	Each test batch New reagent batch	Weak example of A/B if antisera specified for subgroup detection
RhD typing	RhD+ and RhD– cells	Each test batch New reagent batch	Weak D/DVI variant if antisera expected to detect these phenotypes. Manual tests, use manufacturer's control reagent also
Other red cell antigens	Apparent single dose expression of appropriate antigen and cells negative for the antigen	Each batch of tests or single test	
Antibody screening	Weak examples of antibodies, e.g. anti-RhD, anti-Fy^a	Each batch of tests	Other specificities may be substituted or included
Antibody identification	Perform auto-control	Each time	
Titrations	Previous sample in parallel. Cells with apparent single dose antigen expression	Each time	Same cells each time, where possible (frozen aliquots)

Table 8.2 Quality control of laboratory equipment

Equipment	Parameter	Minimum frequency
Refrigerators	Recorder Temperature Alarm activation system (if in place)	Daily Daily Quarterly
Freezers	As above	As above
Incubators	Temperature	Daily
Centrifuges	Speed Timer	Quarterly Quarterly
Cell washers	Saline volume Function	Daily Monthly
Heating blocks/ water baths	Temperature	Daily
Component thawing devices		Daily
pH meters	High and low controls	At time of use
Blood irradiators	Calibration Timer Source decay Dose delivery	Yearly Monthly Dependent on source type Yearly
Thermometers		Yearly
Timers/clocks		Yearly
Pipettes	Calibration Cleaning/decontamination	Yearly Each time of use
Reagent dispensers		Daily
Balances/scales		At time of use

Note: this list is not exhaustive. Any piece of equipment used during the laboratory procedure/process must be tested for functionality at appropriate intervals.

routine laboratory procedures and for laboratory equipment. In order to ensure best practice, quality control, quality assurance and continuous quality improvement in the laboratory include the review and approval of:
- procedures and policies;
- training/education;

- validation of protocols and results;
- calibration of equipment;
- document control/record keeping;
- product specifications;
- suppliers;
- corrective action planning/monitoring;
- error reports;
- health and safety issues (including waste management);
- audits;
- SOPs;
- analysis of trends;
- problem solving;
- external QA results; and
- accreditation issues.

Quality requirements for safe transfusion practice

- The responsibilities of all personnel involved in the transfusion process should be clear and each individual notified.
- Pre-labelled tubes for patients' samples should not be used.
- Samples for pre-transfusion compatibility procedures should be stored at 4–6°C and taken 24 hours before transfusion if a previous transfusion has been administered within the previous 3–14 days. A sample no older than 72 hours may be used if the last transfusion was 14–28 days previously.
- Positive patient identification at sampling and at the time of transfusion is essential for both inpatients and outpatients.
- The request system should ensure prescription issue of blood and/or components and needs to include procedures to ensure the correct administration of the component. Written policies for the collection of components are essential.
- Emergency issue, special requirements, or telephone requests should also be covered in the regulations.
- Laboratories should have access to previous transfusion records including historical grouping and screening results.
- Transfusion committees can help to monitor the efficiency of the procedures and recommend changes where necessary.
- Multi-disciplinary audits of the transfusion process on a regular basis.
- Continuous training of all staff involved in the transfusion chain to ensure compliance with procedures.

Checklist of critical control points

Sample receipt/ acceptance	Patient details match on transfusion request form and sample	Any doubts (e.g. illegible handwriting) new sample to be requested
Patient details entered	Check that the information is correct (spelling, date of birth, hospital number)	Take care about patients with common or similar names
Laboratory tests	Perform as in appropriate SOPs. Enter details	If previously tested, check that results match exactly. Check history of previous transfusions/ pregnancies, previous antibodies
Units for transfusion	Check ABO group/ blood group label	Check component is correct (e.g. irradiated, CMV-negative, etc.)
	Compatibility label after negative cross-match	Check and enter details. Transfer to storage (laboratory/theatre refrigerator, etc.)
Blood collection	Follow established SOP. Recipient identity, signature of individual taking units, etc.	Retain samples post-transfusion. Sample from unit after transfusion essential for investigation of adverse events
Blood administration	Bedside check as per SOP	Monitor patient
Blood return	Establish the unit's suitability to be returned to stock	If accepted, remove compatibility label. Log return details

Laboratory errors, root cause analysis (RCA) and corrective and preventative action (CAPA)

The purpose of pre-transfusion testing is to ensure that the right component of blood is selected and administered to the right patient. This involves many laboratory protocols where errors can and, unfortunately, do occur.

Errors can occur at any time from the point of the tests being ordered to the final reporting of the results and therefore include errors of interpretation and/or errors involving technical or clerical issues.

Laboratory errors can result in the wrong blood being issued and/or transfused. If the wrong sample is tested, the subsequent events can be serious, such as a haemolytic transfusion reaction. Other errors may involve handing or storage, or be associated with different aspects of pre-transfusion testing. For example, the correct sample may be selected and tested but incorrect results recorded. Procedural errors involve the incorrect test selection, resulting in wrong, inadequate, or inappropriate information being recorded.

Some errors can be due to lack of training or experience. For example, recognition of mixed-field (double-cell populations) reactions can be important in preventing a wrong group being assigned. Manual techniques are more prone to errors than automated procedures, so it is recommended to install automated testing with good computer back-up where possible. Training remains imperative, including understanding the equipment and software to be able to utilise the technology most effectively.

Every laboratory must have an established internal incident reporting system as part of TQM. This can include the use of root cause analysis (RCA) techniques when an error is detected. This entails asking questions until the root cause is determined. What happened? How? Why? What are the consequences? Answers should be compared with the established policies and procedures. In other words, what *should* have happened. The 'fishbone' diagram (Fig. 8.1) can be a good starting point to establish where the shortcomings are and/or where errors may originate. Patient factors can include the medication interfering with results, staff factors may highlight physical or even psychological issues. Task-based errors may be due to incorrect SOPs and communication problems can be verbal, written, or electronic and need to be reviewed as part of RCA. If team roles are not well-defined or understood, it could cause an error to occur due to lack of leadership. Other issues should be regularly reviewed during RCA to ensure that the appropriate education and training has been undertaken, that all equipment and resources necessary are available and properly maintained. Working conditions have been shown to contribute

Root Cause Analysis: what happened, where, why, who, how?

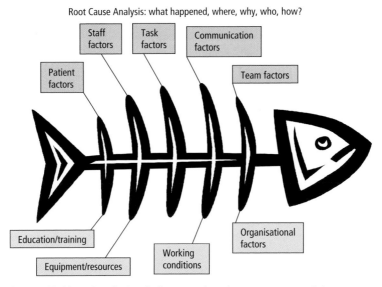

Fig. 8.1 'Fishbone' analysis to help categorise where errors may originate.

to error rates, as it has been shown that errors often occur out of normal working hours. Organisational factors include problems associated with staffing levels and other administrative details but, in general, when an error occurs, it has many contributory elements and may not be due to a single factor.

When the reason(s) for the error has been determined, then corrective and preventative action (CAPA) should be implemented. A process map indicating the step-by-step details can be helpful in analysing what should be changed, how and when a change should be implemented, and by whom.

This type of cause and effect analysis, followed by the appropriate corrective actions will defend against possible error-prone acts or omissions, making each procedure as fool-proof as possible, aiming for zero errors and safe transfusion.

Trouble-shooting and problem-solving in the reference laboratory

CHAPTER 9

ABO grouping

ABO groups should be assigned only when the forward and reverse groupings concur and when the group obtained is identical to either historical records or the results of a second ABO test. However, sometimes discrepancies occur, which must be resolved, often requiring further investigation at a reference laboratory (Fig. 9.1). Prior to referring samples for intensive investigation at a reference laboratory, the laboratory should try to resolve any anomalous results by reviewing areas where a discrepancy may have occurred. Table 9.1 outlines a checklist for helping to resolve ABO discrepancies.

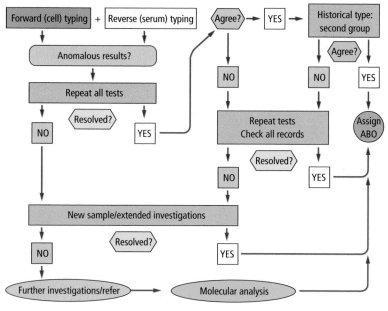

Fig. 9.1 Flow chart for helping to resolve ABO typing discrepancies.

Essential Guide to Blood Groups, 2nd edition. By Geoff Daniels and Imelda Bromilow. Published 2010 by Blackwell Publishing Ltd.

Table 9.1 Guide to resolving ABO discrepancies

Category	Check	
1 General points	• Clerical details • Previous records (transfusion history, medication, age, clinical and obstetric data) • Sample (haemolysed, spontaneous agglutination, lipaemic) • Functionality of reagents/reagent contamination	
2 Preliminary investigations	• Centrifuge sample	
	• Repeat test	Cells and serum Fresh sample Fresh reagents
3 Further techniques	• Patient/donor cells	Wash and repeat
	• Patient/donor serum	Longer incubation time incubate at 4°C
4 Unresolved forward (cell) group discrepancy	If unrelated to age, disease state, or rouleaux formation:	
I *Weak/negative reactions*	• Possible subgroup	Absorption-elution Saliva studies (if secretor) Serum transferase DNA analysis
II *Mixed-field reactions*	If unrelated to transfusion/transplant therapy:	
	• Possible subgroup	See above
	• Possible chimera	Separate cell populations and retest each one
III *Unexpected positive reactions*	• Polyagglutinability of cells	Use of monoclonal sera Lectins to characterise polyagglutination type
	• Direct antiglobulin test (DAT) positive	Remove *in vivo* coating (warm washing cells or other method)
	• Acquired-B phenotype	Check diagnosis Use monoclonal anti-B known not to react
	• Spontaneous agglutination (if sample stored at 4°C prior to test)	Cold autoantibody Retest at 37°C (new sample taken and maintained at 37°C may be necessary)
	• Possible B(A) phenotype	Use other sera

(*Continued*)

Table 9.1 (*Continued*)

Category	Check	
5 Unresolved reverse group discrepancy	If unrelated to age (newborn/elderly), immunosuppression, hypogammaglobulinaemia or haemolysis of the reagent cells consider:	
I *Weak/negative reactions*	• Fresh sample	Retest at 4°C Increase incubation time Use fresh set of cells and/or additional cells Retest forward group for confirmation
II *Additional unexpected reactions*	• Possible alloantibody	Identify specificity Retest with appropriate cells but negative for the corresponding antigen
	• Possible cold autoantibody	Autologus control Use a pre-warmed technique Autoadsorption and retest
	• Possible rouleaux	Saline replacement technique
	• A_2 or lower A subgroups	Reaction with A_1 cells

Notes

1 Recommended laboratory procedures/techniques should be followed for the investigation of any discrepancy (e.g. AABB Technical Manual, other practically based text book, or in-house established standard operating procedures).
2 Where anomalous results persist, family studies can be useful, with serological and molecular biology techniques to establish inheritance pattern and genetic background.
3 This chart is not necessarily comprehensive.

Rh grouping

The basic RhD type should only be assigned when the results of testing, preferentially with two matched monoclonal anti-D sera, are the same and that the D type concurs with historical data available (Fig. 9.2), or according to local or national guidelines for D typing of donors and patients. Rh typing anomalies may be resolved by reviewing areas where a discrepancy may have occurred before referring the sample for further investigation as outlined in Table 9.2.

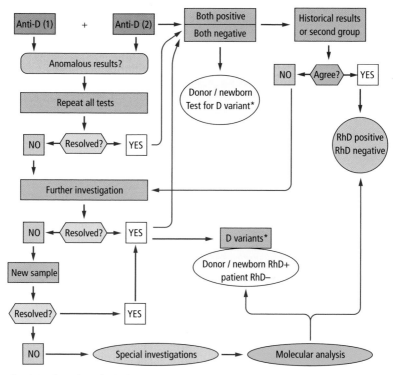

Fig. 9.2 Flow chart for helping to resolve Rh typing discrepancies. Always refer to the relevant local or national guidelines, as recommendations for D typing may vary from this schematic. For example, some countries allow for only one anti-D, some countries require DVI/weak D to be detected in neonatal samples and some countries may require indirect antiglobulin test anti-D typing for donor bloods.

Table 9.2 Guide to resolving Rh discrepancies

Category	Check/control/investigate	
1 **General points**	• Clerical details • Previous records (transfusion history, medication, age, clinical and obstetric data) • Sample (haemolysed, spontaneous coagulation, lipaemic) • Functionality of reagents/reagent contamination	
2 **Preliminary investigations**	• Centrifuge sample	Wash cells
	• Repeat test	Fresh sample Fresh reagents Additional sera of same specificity

(*Continued*)

Table 9.2 (*Continued*)

Category	Check/control/investigate	
3 Unresolved problems		
I *Unexpected positive reactions*	• Check for rouleaux formation related to disease state (rouleaux not associated with gel test systems)	
a Previously tested negative or autocontrol also positive	• Cells DAT positive	Try monoclonal sera Remove *in vivo* coating by warm-washing cells or other approved method
	• Confirm positive result	Adsorption and elution
	• Antibody to low frequency antigen in human antiserum	Use monoclonal antiserum
	• Cells polyagglutinable	Use monoclonal antiserum Lectins to characterise polyagglutination type
	• Sample mix up this time/previous time tested	Check all previous records; confirm identity and repeat from a second sample
b Alloantibody of apparently the same specificity present or positive with one reagent, negative with another of same specificity	• Possible antigen variant – most commonly associated with the D antigen	Test with a panel of anti-D sera to characterise the D variant type Antisera to known Rh low-frequency antigens associated with D variants Family studies Refer to reference laboratory for molecular basis
II *Unexpected weak or negative reactions*	• Weak positive may be due to any reason above. Check and control	
	• Rare phenotypes	Rh_{null}/Rh_{mod} Deletions, e.g. D–– Suppressed antigenic complexes, e.g. D(C)(e)

(*Continued*)

Table 9.2 (*Continued*)

Category	Check/control/investigate	
	• Compound antisera	Human anti-C is most often anti-C + -Ce. Weak or negative reactions with certain phenotypes
	• Sample mix up this time/previous time tested	Check all previous records; confirm identity and repeat from a second sample
III *Mixed-field reactions*	• Post-transfusion	Check records
	• Post-transplantation therapy (bone marrow/ stem cells)	Check records
	• Rh mosaism due to myelo-proliferative disorder	Monitor Rh type beyond remission
	• Chimerism (twin or dispermic)	Separate cell populations and retest Full blood group phenotyping to check for chimerism in other blood group systems Cytogenetic studies Tissue culture, e.g. analysis of fibroblasts

Notes

1 Generally a sample confirmed as a D variant can be treated as RhD positive for donor purposes. Transfusion recipients or antenatal patients should only be treated as RhD positive when clear-cut reactions have been obtained with suitable anti-D reagents in accordance with local or national guidelines.

2 The DVI phenotype is the most important variant to consider.
   • Anti-D known to react with DVI should be used for RhD typing of donor bloods, and weak-D types *should* be detected.
   • Anti-D known *not* to react with DVI bloods should be used for RhD typing of transfusion recipients or antenatal patients.

3 Human anti-D sera most often require a potentiating medium and will give positive reactions with D variants. Care should be exercised not to misclassify a DVI patient sample as RhD positive, particularly in the case of pre-menopausal females.

4 Recommended laboratory procedures and techniques should be followed for the investigation of any discrepancy (e.g. AABB Technical Manual, other practically based textbook, or in-house established standard operating procedures).

5 Where anomalous results persist, family studies can be useful, with serological and molecular biology techniques to establish inheritance pattern and genetic background.

6 This chart is not necessarily comprehensive.

Problems in antibody screening, identification, and cross-matching

In general, problems are encountered when seemingly anomalous results are observed, such as when the antibody is to a low frequency antigen, a high frequency antigen, a mixture of antibodies, due to 'non-specific' antibody, autoantibody, or interference in tests after administration of prophylactic anti-D. Table 9.3 outlines these situations and possible observations regarding test results in order to resolve such difficulties. Table 9.4 outlines some additional information regarding original reactions by indirect antiglobulin test and further investigations that can be considered in order to determine antibody specificity. Some antibodies may be characterised based on reactions with papain-treated red cells in parallel with dithiothreitol treatment as shown in Table 9.5. Reference laboratories may perform additional tests in order to identify or confirm the presence of antibodies such as by the use of cord cells, lacking or having weak expression of certain antigens, or by the use of human body fluids known to neutralise certain antibodies. However, this is beyond the scope of this book.

Table 9.3 Some common problems and observations in antibody investigations

Antibody type	Possible observation	Comments
1 Low frequency antigen	Negative antibody screen, positive cross-match	Compatible blood easily found
2 High frequency antigen	All or most screening and panel cells positive. Autocontrol negative	Compatible blood difficult to find. Test relatives; consider autologous donation; consult national or international rare donor registry
3 Multiple specificities	Varying strength of reactions, most screening and panel cells positive	Confirm each specificity. Phenotype cells. Depending on specificities, compatible blood may be difficult to obtain
4 Post-prophylactic anti-D administration	Anti-D due to antenatal or postnatal administration	RhD negative cells to screen for other antibodies. Passively acquired anti-D will decrease, half-life 21 days. Generally not detected by IAT after 12 weeks

(Continued)

Table 9.3 (*Continued*)

Antibody type	Possible observation	Comments
5 'Non-specific' or non-red cell immune	Positive reactions with no definable pattern	Antibody showing dosage. Cold antibody with high thermal amplitude. Antibody to white cell antigens, expressed on the red cell. Apparent specificity, e.g. anti-E, -K post-infection
6 Autoantibody	All reagent cells positive, plus autocontrol. Sometimes stronger reaction with own cells. DAT positive	Determination of presence of underlying alloantibody important (auto/allo-absorption) Strong 'cold' autoantibody, perform tests at 37°C. Patient history/medication (diagnosis/ drug-dependent condition)
7 Other	a Masked antibodies b 'Positive' reactions due to rouleaux in tube techniques c Haemolysis of reagent cells d Mixed-field (double population) type reactions	a Even if apparent single antibody, always check b Myeloma patients. Dispersed with saline. Not usually seen in column agglutination techniques c May be mistaken for negative reaction in tube techniques. d Characteristic of certain antibodies, e.g. anti-Lu^a, anti-Sd^a Due to use of pooled cells (donor testing only)

DAT, direct antiglobulin test; IAT, indirect antiglobulin test.

Table 9.4 Reaction patterns and tests for the determination of antibody specificity

Results by IAT	Suspect	Useful tests	Further investigations
All + (same strength) Auto negative	HFA	ETC. Other temperatures	HFA-negative cells Masked antibody difficult to demonstrate Include A_1, A_2 cells to exclude anti-HI or anti-Le^{bH} Phenotype patient
All + (different strengths) Auto negative	Mixture	ETC. Other temperatures Check for dosage effect. Check for unlisted antigens	Test for individual antibodies with selected cells Separate IgG and IgM antibodies (DTT/2ME*) Phenotype patient
Some + (same strength) Auto negative	Single antibody	ETC Check for underlying masked antibody	Check for dosage if no specificity found. Phenotype patient
Some + (different strengths) Auto negative	Antigens with different level of expression; antibody showing dosage; Knops system, Cs^a and other, 'nebulous or non-specific' antibodies	Check reactions against cells for dosage/expression Check for Knops system antibodies Check for white blood cell antibody, e.g. anti-Bg specificities	Check for unlisted antigens and/or LFA See Table 9.2 for specialized tests and investigations

HFA, high frequency antigen; ETC, enzyme-treated cells; Ig, immunoglobulin; LFA, low frequency antigen.
* Sulphydryl compounds Dithiothreitol and 2-mercaptoethanol cleave disulphide bonds that join the units of an IgM pentamer. This is useful in antibody mixtures of different immunoglobulin classes, to demonstrate potentially clinically important IgG antibody.

Table 9.5 Further tests for antibody determination

Antibody	Papain-treated cells	DTT (200 mmol)	Remarks
M, N, S, s, Ge2, Ge4, Xg^a, Fy^a, Fy^b, Ch/Rg	Negative	Positive	Anti-s variable with papain Ch/Rg inhibited by plasma/serum. Cord cells Ch/Rg negative
Indian, JMH	Negative	Negative	
Cromer, Knops	Positive	Weak	Cromer antigens on DAF,* therefore absent from PNH† cells
Yt^a	Variable	Negative	Cord cells weak expression
Lutheran, Dombrock,	Positive	Weak	Cord cells weak for Lu^a, Lu^b antigens
Kell, LW, Scianna, MER2	Positive	Negative	Cord cells strong for LW Scianna may be more resistant at lower concentrations of DTT
A, B, H, P1, Lewis, Kidd, Fy3, Diego, Colton, AnWj, Ge3, Ii, P, Cs^a, Vel, Sd^a	Positive	Positive	Cord cells negative for Lewis, strong i ABH, Lewis inhibited by saliva, serum/plasma. Sd^a inhibited by urine (guinea-pig)
Kx	Positive	Enhanced	Antibody made by McLeod phenotype males with CGD‡

*DAF, decay accelerating factor or CD55.

† Paroxysmal nocturnal haemoglobinuria (PNH) is a defect in which red cells lack DAF and membrane inhibitor of reactive lysis (MIRL or CD59) and are sensitive to complement.

‡ Chronic granulomatous disease. The red cells from patients lack the Kx antigen due to deletion of part of the X chromosome. The McLeod phenotype exhibits greatly reduced expression of Kell antigens (see Chapter 5).

Frequently asked questions

CHAPTER 10

What is the difference between sensitivity and specificity and how can these be determined?

Sensitivity is the number of positive results obtained, in comparison with the number of truly positive samples. Specificity is the number of negative results in comparison with truly negative samples. Evaluation is carried out against the 'gold standard' test. Care must be exercised to ensure that the 'gold standard' is actually the most accurate and efficient method prior to making comparisons.

		Test 1		
		Positive	Negative	
Test 2	Positive	A	B	A+B
	Negative	C	D	C+D
Total		A+C	B+D	A+B+C+D

Sensitivity = A/A+C
Specificity = D/B+D

Why is anti-A,B no longer obligatory in ABO typing?

Anti-A,B was used to help in the detection of subgroups of A and B when only human polyclonal antisera was available. It is now generally accepted that for routine blood grouping, monoclonal anti-A and -B reagents are sufficiently potent to detect such subgroups alone. Similarly, recommendations for reverse grouping have been reduced to A_1 and B cells only. Some examples of low subgroups (e.g. A_x, A_m) may not be

---

Essential Guide to Blood Groups, 2nd edition. By Geoff Daniels and Imelda Bromilow. Published 2010 by Blackwell Publishing Ltd.

recognised using this format, but clinically this is not considered important. An A_x or A_m transfusion recipient could safely receive group O red cells. However, an A subgroup would be indicated by the reverse (serum/plasma) grouping test not being in accordance with a 'group O' forward (cell) typing and would be fully investigated.

Why are two anti-D sera often recommended for RhD typing?

The second test acts as a control against reagent malfunction or other technical errors. In ABO typing, the reverse grouping serves as a control for the forward (cell) typing, but this needs to be achieved by the use of a second reagent in the case of RhD status determination.

What is the importance of detecting D variant (weak D and partial D) phenotypes?

In donors, a D variant (weak D or partial D) phenotype should mean that the unit is labelled as RhD positive. This is to prevent D variant cells being transfused to a recipient who is RhD negative, with the consequence that the recipient could produce an anti-D in response (although there is debate about the immunogenicity of D variant red cells with very weak expression of D).

It is generally considered safer to treat antenatal patients and potential transfusion recipients as RhD negative, even when their true Rh type is a D variant. This is because they will be transfused with RhD negative blood, which is acceptable, although considered by some workers as a waste of RhD negative blood. Antenatal patients will receive prophylactic anti-D, but this is not considered harmful. Again, it might be thought to be wasteful of a precious resource, plus it means exposing women to unnecessary blood products.

Neonatal RhD typing does not require the detection of D variants and anti-D reagents should be chosen accordingly. There is little evidence that such cells provoke the production of anti-D in the maternal circulation.

How do I control the results for antiglobulin testing?

In spin-tube antiglobulin testing, a leading cause of false negative results is due to a poor wash phase, after which residual human proteins not removed from the test system neutralise the anti-human globulin (AHG). In order to check the validity of a negative antiglobulin spin-tube test, it is necessary to add sensitised control cells to the completed test. If the AHG has not been neutralised, the test should become positive and a negative result for the sample may be designated. If the control cells fail to agglutinate, the test is invalid and should be repeated, ensuring that the wash phase is properly carried out. The control cells should be *weakly* sensitised for maximum sensitivity of the test.

In gel technology, antiglobulin tests are not required to be washed and therefore this control is not required.

Why should RhD positive women be tested more than once during pregnancy?

RhD positive women can make anti-c, a leading cause of haemolytic disease of the fetus and newborn (HDFN). Other antibodies known to be implicated in the disease can be made by any woman, regardless of Rh phenotype, for example anti-K. Also, a second or subsequent check of ABO and RhD status acts as a control for the first determination and may reveal errors previously unnoticed (e.g. wrong sample or misinterpretation of original results).

How often should transfusion recipients be tested for the presence of antibodies?

Most European guidelines recommend the following:

Last transfused within:	Sample to be taken:
3–14 days	24 hours before transfusion
14–28 days	72 hours before transfusion
28 days to 3 months	1 week before transfusion

In the USA, a sample must be taken within 72 hours for patients transfused within the 3-month period.

How can passive anti-D be differentiated from anti-D due to alloimmunisation?

In general, this is not possible in routine testing situations. The half-life of immunoglobulin G (IgG) is about 23–26 days and therefore the strength of reactions with RhD positive cells and values obtained in quantification procedures will decrease over time, with passive anti-D. Known administration of anti-D antenatally can interfere with screening for other alloantibodies and a set of cells negative for the D antigen, but positive in double-dose for other important antigens, may be included in the investigations of such samples.

Why do we need to perform antibody screening? Isn't a cross-match by indirect antiglobulin test at 37°C enough to detect incompatible blood?

Screening identifies patients with antibodies prior to cross-matching, so that antigen-negative blood can be selected for cross-matching. An antibody screen uses 'matched' sets of 2, 3, or 4 cells that possess all the relevant antigens in double-dose, making the likelihood of detecting a clinically important antibody high. The spread of available antigens is also greater with a set of screening cells and account can be taken of population differences where appropriate (e.g. Di^a, Mur). A subsequent cross-match may be positive due to the presence of a low frequency antigen on the donor cells lacking from the screening cells. However, a negative cross-match does not mean that the recipient does not possess an antibody of potential importance. It may be that the antibody shows 'dosage' and will not react *in vitro* with the donor cells, but can still be capable of initiating accelerated destruction of the transfused cells *in vivo*.

What is the incidence of alloimmunisation post-transfusion?

About 2–10% in general. Antibodies most often found are to E, K, c, Fy^a, Kidd, Lewis, s, and S. Patients with pre-existing antibodies are at a 3–4 times higher risk of developing further antibodies.

How do I determine and identify antibodies present in a sample?

Using the 'rule out' method, eliminate any antigen that possesses a double-dose where a negative result has been observed. Antigens not eliminated in this way are then evaluated. A full phenotype of the patient will reveal which antibodies the person can make. The reaction method can also help, for example where an antibody is directed against an enzyme sensitive antigen. Sometimes, extended and/or special techniques may be required, or the determination of separate antibodies may need to be undertaken at a reference centre. Cells are selected that are negative for all possibilities but one, for each suspected specificity, until the antibody is confirmed or not. For example, a mixture suspected to be anti-M, $-Fy^a$, and -S requires cells that are M+ N–, Fy(a–b+), S– s+; M– N+, Fy(a+b–), S– s+; and M– N+, Fy(a–b+), S+ s–. Confirmation of each specificity requires reactivity with at least two examples of reagent red cells carrying the appropriate antigen and non-reactivity with at least two cells lacking the antigen.

What is a compound antibody?

A compound antibody is one that only reacts with red cells possessing more than one specificity encoded by the same gene. The most well-known are to be found within the Rh system. Anti-f is a compound antibody directed against cells with c and e antigens, carried on the same protein; that is, anti-f will react with cells of the phenotype DCe/d<u>ce</u> but not with DCe/DCe or DC<u>e</u>/D<u>c</u>E.

How can the incidence of compatible donors for a recipient with multiple antibodies be calculated?

Multiply the antigen negative incidence for each antibody specificity (taking into account any population differences as necessary):

for example, anti-K + -Jk^a + -S

K negative incidence = 0.91 (Causcasian population)

Jk^a negative incidence = 0.23

S negative incidence = 0.48

0.91 × 0.23 × 0.48 = 0.10 or 1 in 10 donors.

If 6 units are required from random donors (not phenotyped) then 60 units would need to be tested.

The ABO and Rh type of the patient have an important role in the ease of providing blood compatible with multiple antibodies. All blood in stock can be tested for a group AB RhD positive patient but group O recipients can only receive group O units. The provision of RhD negative blood is most important for RhD negative women of child-bearing age.

Why can't the droppers in bottles of reagents be used instead of a volumetric pipette?

Droppers in bottles of reagents, in common with glass or plastic pipettes, are not calibrated for accurately dispensing a given volume of reagent. The volume dispensed can alter radically with the pressure applied to the bulb and/or the angle at which the dropper/pipette is held. Certain test systems require the serum : cell ratio to be within defined limits, which will not be respected if using an inaccurate means of dispensing reagents. For example, for low ionic strength saline antiglobulin tests, the serum : cell ratio should be a minimum of 40 : 1. The serum : cell ratio of a technique may be established using the formula:

$$\frac{\text{Volume serum} \times 100}{\text{Volume red blood cell (RBC)} \times (\% \text{ concentration})}$$

What is 'massive transfusion'?

Massive transfusion is arbitrarily defined as the replacement of a patient's total blood volume in less than 24 hours, or as the acute administration of more than half of the patient's estimated blood volume per hour. For transfusion, ABO group identical blood is the first choice and may be administered without serological cross-matching. ABO incompatibility must be excluded. Where ABO identical blood is not available, blood of the same group as the patient should be used as soon as possible. It is not necessary to continue with the ABO group originally selected.

When group-specific blood is in short supply, how do I select the 'next best' for transfusion?

For group AB patients the second choice should be group A or B red cells to conserve stocks of group O blood. For patients of group A or B, the second choice should be group O, provided that it is plasma depleted or does not contain high-titre haemagglutinins. RhD positive blood may be administered to RhD negative recipients, except for women under 60 years of age.

How are high-titre haemagglutinins classified?

In Europe and Asia, they are generally defined as an IgM >1 : 32 to >1 : 100 or an IgG >1 : 256 to 1 : 512. In the USA, the definition is IgM >1 : 50 to 1 : 64 and/or IgG >256. However, it must be noted that components from group O donors with 'low titres' of anti-A, -B, and/or -A,B can cause intravascular haemolysis in non-group O recipients if given in large volumes.

What is an 'immediate spin' cross-match?

The immediate spin (IS) technique is used to provide assurance that the donor unit is ABO compatible with the recipient's blood. The recommended technique is a 2 : 1 ratio of serum/plasma to cells suspended in ethylenediaminetetraacetic acid (EDTA) saline, at a concentration of 2–3%. An incubation of 2–5 minutes at room temperature enhances the detection of weak ABO antibodies.

What is an 'electronic cross-match'?

This is when no serological cross-matching is performed, but blood of the correct ABO/D type is identified for a patient within the hospital computer system. If the patient requires transfusion, the allocated units can be issued and withdrawn for use. To implement electronic issue, the antibody screening methods and the computer system must conform to current guidelines. Standard operating procedures for the checking of units collected and transfused must be conformed to.

Which patients are not eligible for electronic issue of blood?

- Patients known to have, or who have had, antibodies of potential clinical importance.
- When the antibody screen in routine use does not conform to recommended procedures with regard to technique or minimum requirements for antigens on the screening cells.
- A patient who has had an ABO-incompatible solid-organ transplant and is being transfused within 3 months of the procedure.

- Fetuses or neonates being transfused for alloimmune disease.
- Care should also be taken if the patient population includes ethnic minority groups, associated with different antigen frequencies than the general population.

What is 'bed-side' testing?

This is a final check of compatibility between the patient and the donor unit, performed immediately before the blood is transfused. This is a serological test that is obligatory in some countries, but not approved of in others. Whether or not this test is implemented, it is imperative that a final check be made at the bed-side to ensure that the correct unit is being administered to the correct patient. Remote checking leads to transfusion errors.

What are signs and symptoms of a suspected transfusion reaction?

Fever of >38°C and increase of at least 1°C from baseline (febrile non-haemolytic reaction, bacterial contamination if rigors/hypotension or acute haemolytic transfusion reaction).

Urticaria (rash due to allergic reaction, anaphylaxis, depending on other symptoms).

Dyspnoea with hypertension (possible circulatory overload) or hypotension (acute haemolytic transfusion reaction, bacterial contamination, transfusion-related acute lung injury).

What action should be taken in the event of a suspected transfusion reaction?

1 Stop transfusion.
2 Keep vein open with saline and a new IV set.
3 Check vital signs.
4 Check that the correct unit has been given to the correct patient.
5 Notify medic in charge.
6 Notify the blood bank.

Where necessary, the donor units should be returned to the blood bank along with blood and urine samples from the patient for investigation.

In haemovigilance, how should 'near-miss' events be characterised?

Most haemovigilance systems have well-defined characteristics for major morbidity as a result of blood transfusion and these systems are increasingly encouraging the reporting of near-miss events. These are events that expose a defect in the security process of the transfusion chain. The near-miss event means that no patient was harmed because the fault was spotted and rectified. Some near-miss events could have led to major morbidity or even the death of the recipient, whereas others may have led to a benign result. However, all should be reported and identified in order to assess the requirement for altering the procedures to avoid the near-miss being repeated, with possible serious consequences.

Recommended reading

Anstee DJ. Red cell genotyping and the future of pretransfusion testing. Blood 2009; 114: 248–256.

Burton NM, Anstee DJ. Nature, function and significance of Rh proteins in red cells. Curr Opin Hematol 2008; 15: 625–630.

Chester AM, Olsson ML. The ABO blood group gene: a locus of considerable genetic diversity. Transfus Med Rev 2001; 15: 177–200.

Coombs RA. Historical note: past, present and future of the antiglobulin test. Vox Sang 1998; 74: 67–73.

Daniels G. Human Blood Groups, 2nd edn. Oxford: Blackwell Science, 2002.

Daniels G. Functions of red cell surface proteins. Vox Sang 2007; 93: 331–340.

Daniels G. The molecular genetics of blood group polymorphism. Hum Genet 2009; 126: 729–742.

Daniels G, Finning K, Martin P, Massey E. Non-invasive prenatal diagnosis of fetal blood group phenotypes: current practice and future prospects. Prenat Diagn 2009; 29: 101–107.

Daniels G and members of the ISBT Working Party on Terminology for Red Cell Surface Antigens. Blood group terminology 2004. Vox Sang 2004; 87: 304–316, updated Vox Sang 2009; 96: 153–156.

Hillyer C, Shaz BH, Winkler AM, Reid M. Integrating molecular technologies for red blood cell typing and compatibility testing into blood centers and transfusion services. Transfus Med Rev 2008; 22: 117–132.

Klein H, Anstee DJ. Mollison's Blood Transfusion in Clinical Medicine, 11th edn. Oxford: Blackwell Science, 2005.

Petz L, Garratty G. Immune Haemolytic Anemias, 2nd edn. Philadelphia: Churchill Livingstone, 2004.

Poole J, Daniels G. Blood group antibodies and their significance in transfusion medicine. Transfus Med Rev 2007; 21: 58–71.

Rabson A, Roitt I, Delves P. Really Essential Medical Immunology, 2nd edn. Oxford: Wiley-Blackwell Science, 2004.

Reid ME, Lomas-Francis CG. Blood Group Antigen Facts Book, 2nd edn. New York: Academic Press, 2003.

Roback JD, Combs MR, Grossman BJ, Hillyer CD (eds). AABB Technical Manual, 16th edn. Maryland: American Association of Blood Banks, 2008.

Westhoff CM. The Rh blood group system in review: a new face for the next decade. Transfusion 2004; 44: 1663–1673.

Yamamoto E. Review: ABO blood group system – ABH oligosaccharide antigens, anti-A and anti-B, A and B glycosyltransferases, and ABO genes. Immuno-hematology 2004; 20: 3–22.

Index

Page numbers in *italics* represent figures, those in **bold** represent tables.